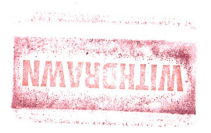

INSIDE DOPE

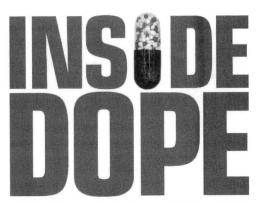

INSIDE DOPE

HOW DRUGS ARE THE BIGGEST THREAT TO SPORTS, WHY YOU SHOULD CARE, AND WHAT CAN BE DONE ABOUT THEM

RICHARD W. POUND

T 30011000155433

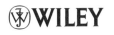 WILEY

John Wiley & Sons Canada, Ltd.

Copyright © 2006 by Richard W. Pound

All rights reserved. No part of this work covered by the copyright herein may be reproduced or used in any form or by any means—graphic, electronic or mechanical—without the prior written permission of the publisher. Any request for photocopying, recording, taping or information storage and retrieval systems of any part of this book shall be directed in writing to The Canadian Copyright Licensing Agency (Access Copyright). For an Access Copyright license, visit www.accesscopyright.ca or call toll free 1-800-893-5777.

Care has been taken to trace ownership of copyright material contained in this book. The publisher will gladly receive any information that will enable them to rectify any reference or credit line in subsequent editions.

National Library of Canada Cataloguing in Publication Data

Pound, Richard W

    Inside dope : How Drugs Are the Biggest Threat to Sports, Why You Should Care, and What Can be Done About Them / Richard W. Pound.

Includes index.

ISBN-13: 978-0-470-83733-7
ISBN-10: 0-470-83733-0

    1. Doping in sports. 2. Athletes—Drug use. I. Title.

RC1230.P69 2006   362.29'088796   C2006-902220-8

Production Credits:
Concept developers and editors: Adrianna Edwards & Ron Edwards,
    Focus Strategic Communications Incorporated
Cover design: Karen Satok
Interior text design: Tegan Wallace
Cover Photo: Tom Schierlitz/Getty Images
Printer: Freisens

John Wiley & Sons Canada, Ltd.
6045 Freemont Blvd.
Mississauga, Ontario
L5R 4J3

Printed in Canada

1 2 3 4 5 FP 10 09 08 07 06

To parents who love their children.
To athletes who love their sport.
To officials with the courage of their convictions.

CONTENTS

Introduction	Who Cares?	1
Chapter 1	Rules Are Not Made to Be Ignored	7
Chapter 2	Winning: At What Price?	19
Chapter 3	What Is Doping?	35
Chapter 4	Test Tube Athletes	51
Chapter 5	Doping Is Not an Accident	67
Chapter 6	Testing: Games People Play	79
Chapter 7	Why Do We Need to Regulate Doping?	91
Chapter 8	Playing Fair, and Willing to Prove It	105
Chapter 9	Pro Sports I: Baseball, Football and Basketball	121
Chapter 10	Pro Sports II: Hockey, Soccer, Golf and Other Sports	145
Chapter 11	Drug Cartels and Drug Pushers in the Wide World of Sport	163
Chapter 12	Gene Doping	179
Chapter 13	See No Evil, Hear No Evil, Speak No Evil	189
Chapter 14	Is There a Cure? My Ten-Step Program	213
Afterword		229
Index		239

INTRODUCTION
WHO CARES?

Who cares about drug use in sport? Let the athletes do whatever they want. It's their bodies, after all, and if they don't care, why should we worry?

How many times have we heard this? I'll bet often enough that it may have an impact on how we think about performance-enhancing drugs and how they have gradually become an ingrained part of sport—the culture of doping. Many believe that drug use simply does not matter. Everybody is doing it. Let the athletes do what they want. The cost of catching the cheaters is too high anyway, so don't waste your money. You will always be a step or two behind the cheaters, so why bother? Why bother with trying to stop doping in the first place?

This attitude is wrong. For one thing, sporting heroes are role models to kids, and do we want our little moppets doing what they see their heroes doing? Not only is it also dangerous to the health of athletes who use drugs—and

INTRODUCTION

not just in mild terms but sometimes fatally—it's most importantly dangerous to the ethics of sport. This attitude is like a disease that can spread beyond the playing fields and have an impact on the entire lives of athletes, those close to them and our society as a whole.

We need to confront this problem. It will not go away on its own. It has already spread to the top amateur and professional athletes. Hardly a week goes by without new revelations. While writing this book during the week of golf's 2006 Masters Tournament, I saw a newspaper report of a sixteen-year-old athlete's suspension for two years as a result of the use of three different prohibited drugs. A sixteen-year-old!

The problem gets worse. We are all familiar with the advances in medical science that have eradicated some diseases or made them treatable. There are many miracle drugs that can manage illnesses and extend life beyond anything we possibly could have imagined, even in the midst of the astonishing technical and scientific progress during our own lifetimes. Almost everyone uses some form of medication. Never in recorded history have so many drugs been available for consumption. There is a pill for practically everything. And now, the genetic codes that distinguish human beings from plankton have been identified, and genes themselves can be manipulated. For the moment, all the known research and clinical trials in gene transfer technology aim to cure terrible diseases like muscular dystrophy. It was the same fifty years ago with the development of modern drugs. Initially, all of them had a therapeutic application.

The difficulty is that a drug that can help someone who is unhealthy can also be used by healthy athletes to gain an "edge" (whether of size, strength or endurance) over other competitors. Unfortunately, the same applies to genetic manipulation. Genes can be altered to produce stronger muscles and to increase delivery of oxygen to the blood and muscles. The practical application of this new technology to sport may be just around the corner. We may see it as early as the 2008 Olympic Games in Beijing. There is no reason to believe that human nature will suddenly change and decide that such procedures will never be used in sport.

There will be scientists who will refuse to be a part of the unethical uses of gene transfer technology, but there will also be those willing to operate outside professional and ethical boundaries with no regard for any rules. Some coaches and athletes are already clamoring to have access to genetic doping techniques, even though they know that the techniques are still very much at the experimental stage. Some coaches have approached scientists to get genetic treatment for their entire teams. The scientists are horrified. They explain that they are still working, experimentally, with rats. They have no idea what might be the effects of their experiments if applied to humans. The coaches don't care. They will accept whatever risks there may be. Besides, in their distorted view, risk is what happens to other people, not to them. I have heard rumors that some individuals have already made attempts. So far, they have not been successful, and, fortunately, no one has died—yet.

So, why should we care about performance-enhancing substances? Well, do we want our children to be forced to become drug addicts in order to be successful in sport? Do we want our children to be in the hands of some unethical scientist or coach, messing with their genes, to bring about some altered creature that we might not even recognize? Every drug and every procedure has side effects, and many of these have not even been identified. Some side effects are irreversible. Too many young athletes around the world are

INTRODUCTION

dying while competing or shortly afterward, or far too early and in greater numbers than they should. Just for starters, here are some recent examples:

- Denis Zanette (Italy) cycling—died January 2003, age 32. Heart attack
- Steve Bechler (U.S.) baseball—died February 2003, age 23. Multi-organ failure
- Marco Ceriani (Italy) cycling—died May 2003, age 16. Heart attack
- Fabrice Salanson (France) cycling—died June 2003, age 23. Heart attack
- Marc-Vivien Foe (Cameroon) soccer—died June 2003, age 28. Heart attack.
- Marco Rusconi (Italy) cycling—died November 2003, age 23. Heart attack
- Jose Maria Jimenez (Spain) cycling—died December 2003, age 32. Heart attack
- Michel Zanoli (Netherlands) cycling—died December 2003, age 35. Heart attack
- Johan Sermon (Belgium) cycling—died February 2004, age 21. Heart attack
- Marco Pantani (Italy) cycling—died February 2004, age 34. Heart attack
- Miklos Feher (Hungary) soccer—died April 2004, age 24. Heart attack
- Alessio Galetti (Italy) cycling—died June 2004, age 34. Heart attack
- David Di Tomasso (France) soccer—died November 2005, age 26. Heart attack

Many of these deaths are directly connected with performance-enhancing drugs, whether or not their presence was detected at the time of death. Do you want your child to be one of these statistics?

On a personal level, apart from needless exposure to the obvious dangers, do we want our children to live a lie, forced to hide what they have done to achieve some degree of ephemeral success in sport? That's not what I want for my kids! Sport is supposed to be fun. It should make you feel better about yourself, not worse.

All of us can—and should—be part of the solution rather than part of the problem. Whether as athlete, parent, coach, trainer, team doctor, sports official, public servant or simply as a member of the public, we must recognize the problem and insist that it be solved. In the end, it's up to us.

So, who cares about doping in sport? Well, I care. So do others. So should you. So should we all.

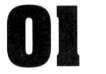 **Rules Are Not
Made to Be Ignored**

If ethics were to disappear from sport, sport will no longer have value as a social and educational tool.

SPORT AND RULES

Sport is part of the games-playing matrix that is peculiar to humans. A lot of animals like to play, but human beings seem to be hardwired for game-playing. It is a fundamental characteristic of the human race.

If, at this moment, all our memories were wiped out and we had no recollection whatsoever of any game or sport, it would probably be a matter of hours before someone would pick up a stone and throw it at another object to see if he could hit it. Or try to run faster than someone else. Or hit an object with a stick. Or lift a heavy weight. Others would try to follow suit to see who could hit closest to the target, run the fastest, bash the object the farthest, lift the heaviest weight.

CHAPTER ONE

Before long, we would agree on rules about how each challenge would be attempted, what was OK and what was not. Games would be developed, with a series of established rules and regulations for each. Someone would eventually write the rules and regulations down so that everyone would know how the game was to be played. Others would agree to act as referees in order to make sure that everyone followed the rules. Competitions would spring up between individuals and groups and, in time, we would get back to where we are right now—with a complex international sports system, involving hundreds of millions of athletes and even more spectators. There would, in all likelihood, be an astonishing similarity to the essential elements of what we now know as sports and games. OK, maybe not cricket or real tennis, but many of the sports we now enjoy.

One of the most important elements of sport is that the participants agree on the rules. Think about it: without the rules, there would be no games. In many respects, these rules are artificial, occasionally arbitrary, but that is not the point. The point is that they are the rules of the game and, furthermore, that they are rules upon which the participants have agreed. If you are competing against me in a game, I expect that you will follow the rules. You are entitled to the same expectations of me.

If all of us who play the game agree to change the rules, for whatever reason, that's fine, but, until we do, neither of us can unilaterally change them. If in the shotput, we decide that the shot will weigh sixteen pounds, I cannot hollow out mine and compete with a twelve-pound shot just because I am not as strong as you, or because your technique is more effective than mine and I need something to "level the playing field" in my eyes. I cannot play hockey with a bigger curve in the stick or use a corked bat in baseball.

I can't start a race before the official signal or run only eleven laps instead of the required twelve. And so on.

The rules are, if you like, our social contract with each other. That's our deal. In society in general, you may be governed by laws with which you may not agree or in which you had no say, but in sport, you always have a choice. If you do not agree with the rules, you do not have to participate. It's quite simple. You are in, or you are out. I'm not going to offer any moral judgment regarding someone who opts out. That is a free choice and a matter of individual decision. But if someone pretends to accept the rules and then cheats, that's something else entirely.

Today, there are lots of rules. Some of them are technical, such as for equipment, size of playing fields, number of players and measurement of success or winning. Some are safety-driven, such as helmets or padding for skiers, hockey players and boxers. Some are designed to protect health, such as minimum ages for competitors, weight categories, medical examinations and safety nets. And so it goes. This is what we buy into when we participate in sport. We promise to play by the rules. It is our ethical commitment, to ourselves and to our opponents and to any spectators who may watch us play.

SPORT AND ETHICS

Thinking outside the box may be a useful way to bring new perspective to problem solving. Playing outside the box of agreed rules for sport is quite another. There may be many motivations for cheating, whether personal glory, insecurity, money, national pride, professional status or a host of others. Whatever they may be, and there is no simple answer to what leads to it, the cheating ruins everything for which sport should stand.

CHAPTER ONE

I have spent some fifty-five years in the Olympic Movement, either as an athlete or official. At its best, I believe the Olympic Movement, with its emphasis on sport and culture, has the potential to provide more for more young people throughout the world—and their countries—than almost anything else I can imagine. The combination of healthy bodies and healthy, inquiring minds that can be developed through sport leads to tremendous personal and societal resources.

A principal reason for the Olympic Movement's potential is that it is based on ethical principles that include self-respect, respect for one's competitors, respect for the rules of play, respect for the officials who ensure that the rules are followed, teamwork, self-discipline, fair play and the renunciation of violence. Each of these values is important in sport, and each is readily transferable to daily participation in society at large. Leaving aside the obvious fact that a healthier society is more productive and cheaper to operate than one that is not, the greater the number of ambitious, goal-setting, competitive, team-working individuals who interact in a particular society, the more vigorous and competitive that society will become.

I believe strongly in these values. They have been important to me throughout my life, and I am convinced that whatever success I may have enjoyed in the things I have done can be traced to those values. Now, I'm not saying that the Olympic values are the *only* set of ethical principles that can lead to a healthy person and a healthy society, but they have the advantage of being relatively simple to understand, and they can be applied to everyone in sport—whether or not they are stars on the field of play. The underlying values are not tied to the level of performance on the field of play, although they are inseparable from the quality of the experience. No matter at what level you may participate

Rules Are Not Made to Be Ignored

(sandlot, intramural, intercollegiate, state, national or international), the experience will be unsatisfactory if other competitors cheat or ignore the concept of fair play.

I don't know about you, but I can accept a loss in a sporting event if someone is better than I am, whether generally or on that particular day. That is all part of the challenge and the excitement of sport—to see who can do the best. There will be days when you win and others when you do not. That is the risk you take when you are a competitor. But the experience can easily be soured when someone cheats.

In my swimming career, where I was fortunate enough to win more often than I lost, a loss was never something I enjoyed. I was trying to win and invested a good deal of time and effort to increase the odds of doing so. But I knew that, from time to time, because someone was better than I was or because I did not prepare adequately or because of a tactical mistake, I would certainly lose.

When someone failed to touch the wall on turns or took off prematurely on a relay exchange, I knew at once, as would everyone, that results achieved that way were unfair. I also played a lot of competitive squash and had the experience soured on many occasions when opponents played double bounces, made bad line calls or interfered to block access to shots. If this type of conduct were allowed to proliferate, sport would lose its meaning and value. If ethics disappear from sport, sport will no longer have value as a social and educational tool.

One of the rules in national and international sport is that doping is prohibited. Doping is the international term that refers to the use of performance-enhancing substances or methods. The original anti-doping rules were adopted out of concerns for the health and safety of the athletes. But, while we're obviously still very much concerned with

CHAPTER ONE

the health of the athletes, the rules have evolved to protect the ethics underlying sport.

The prohibited substances and methods of doping have varied over time with the expansion of scientific know-ledge. A few have been removed from the list of prohibited substances and methods or reclassified for purposes of further study. Others have been added as scientists have become aware of the effects and side effects of their use. What is on or off the list from time to time is not particularly important from a conceptual perspective. What *is* important is that we all agree that we will not use or do the things that are on the list. That, as I have said, is our deal with each other. Our promise to each other.

We are not perfect, though, and there are those who are quite willing to ignore rules to get an unfair advantage over their competitors. Cheaters are the sociopaths of sport, who care nothing for their own promises, who do not respect their fellow competitors, who do not respect the game they are playing and who, in the end, do not even respect themselves. All that matters to them is winning at any cost, and they are willing to cheat or willing to be persuaded to cheat in order to win.

Based on my experience in the field, I have concluded that, in most cases, it is not athletes acting alone. They are assisted, counseled, sometimes tricked and occasionally forced into cheating. Coaches, trainers, medical doctors, scientists, sports administrators, agents, international or national sports federations, national Olympic committees and even some misguided parents (all of whom know better or who have a professional or moral responsibility to the young people under their charge) conspire to destroy the value of what the athletes are trying to do. Some of the worst offenders in the past have been governments, whose distorted sense of national pride has led them to achieve results by organized cheating.

Why should athletes—your children, your neighbors' children or anyone's children—be forced into the downward cycle of the lowest common denominator simply because there are some who are willing to cheat, with all of the risks of disgrace and health problems that may follow? There is an easy answer to this question. They should not.

And here is where the need to ensure a level playing field comes in. Someone must act to protect those who play fair. It is important to develop a culture focused on the prevention of cheating, creating a new mind-set and helping everyone involved to understand the reasons why there should be no cheating. It is also important to be realistic. In society, there will always be those who act outside the law, which is why we have police forces, court systems and specified punishments for breaking the law. It would be foolish to think that similar mechanisms are not required in sport.

CHEATING IS WRONG. PERIOD.

There are no shades of gray when it comes to cheating. Either you are playing fair or you are not.

Athletes who cheat destroy the whole purpose of what they set out to do: to see how far their natural talents—honed by practice to improve skills, strategies and conditioning—can take them in competition with others, playing by the rules. Instead of something that should be a triumph of the human spirit, their achievements become dirty and must be hidden for fear of exposure and disgrace. The image that always comes to my mind in these circumstances is

CHAPTER ONE

that of Oscar Wilde's *The Picture of Dorian Gray*, where the public façade of respectability was contrasted so starkly by the hidden portrait that showed the increasingly disgusting reality of Gray's character.

The officials who cheat make a mockery of their responsibilities and trivialize the years of training and dedication of the trusting athletes whom they betray. A notorious example of corrupt judging occurred at the Salt Lake City Olympic Winter Games in 2002, when French and Russian officials conspired to fix the results in the pairs figure skating event. Canadians Jamie Salé and David Pelletier were betrayed by figure skating officials and judges who were fixing results to further personal ambitions. This happens all too often, and not just in figure skating.

Medical doctors and scientists conspire to assist athletes and others to cheat by developing and administering performance-enhancing drugs. They know that what they are doing is against the rules of sport and that the drugs are potentially harmful to the athletes who use them. In many cases, the side effects are little known, yet they risk the health of athletes because they want to win. The designer steroid THG went directly from the laboratory into the systems of athlete users. The Hippocratic oath, sworn by all medical doctors, includes the undertaking to do no harm. Do no harm, indeed!

And as for coaches, in my view, there is no coach worthy of the description who can be unaware of drug use by athletes under her or his care. It is a responsibility of coaches to develop—and not to destroy—the health and character of those under their care. I do not want my children or grandchildren under the influence of a coach willing to encourage or permit them to use drugs. The role of the coach is not simply to produce better athletic performance, but to develop the athlete as a complete human being.

Rules Are Not Made to Be Ignored

We have not been sufficiently stringent in pursuing the coaches of athletes who use performance-enhancing drugs. That is going to change.

One of our missions at the World Anti-Doping Agency (WADA), which I chair, is to make sure that it is not only the athletes who are punished for doping offences. Often they are less to blame than the coaches, doctors and others around them. A year or so ago, the IOC Athletes' Commission suggested that doping control forms, signed by athletes when they are tested, include spaces to add the names of the athlete's coach and doctor. Then, in case of a positive result, all three may be liable. This suggestion has since been adopted by WADA.

Because much of this is a work in progress, there is little doubt that there will be new revelations even between the time this book goes to press and when it hits the bookshelves. I certainly do not expect that there will be an instant cure for the problem of doping in sport. There is no magic bullet. It will take years to get to where I hope we can reach.

For me, however, one of the main challenges is to not let anything dull the sharp edges of the problem. Doping is cheating and, in many cases, dangerous cheating. It has no place in sport. The sport rules must be applied to protect the overwhelming majority of athletes who play fairly. Cheaters cannot be allowed to go on cheating. If you listen to what is said in public, you can identify the interests that are being served by the efforts to subtly direct arguments in favor of doping, to excuse it, to deny its existence or to pretend that it does not matter. By far the greatest misdirection comes from those who have been caught and from those paid to defend such improper conduct. I will give some examples in Chapter 8 ("Playing Fair, and Willing to Prove It") to illustrate this point.

CHAPTER ONE

Technically, doping in sport is not a criminal activity (depending on the substances), but rather one that should be handled within the sport context, as a breach of a sport rule, and where necessary with the help of governments. The World Anti-Doping Agency is attempting to level the playing field. It performs an absolutely independent role in trying to make sport doping-free. We bring together the sports movement and the governments of the world and put them at the same table, at the same time, with the same objective: to restore the integrity of sport by giving every athlete an equal chance of doing his or her best without having to cheat. In Chapter 7, I describe how WADA came into existence and how it introduced a new dynamic in the fight against doping in sport.

Those of us in a position to help prepare our youth for useful roles in society have a duty to do whatever we can to ensure that our guidance is positive. To win their confidence, we need to show them that the values we talk about are the same values that we practice, support and protect for their benefit. It is a huge responsibility, particularly in a world that is struggling to find its way, and in which the remarkable pace of change has produced an unfortunate tendency to believe that whatever may come from the past is *passé* and of no value.

There is nothing *passé* about trying to do your best, within the limits we must all accept as members of civilized society, whether on the field of play in sport, or on the general field of play within society. There is nothing *passé* about ethical principles, about respect for yourself and for others. We should embrace the positive values of understanding who we are, doing what is morally right and rejecting what is morally wrong—not because someone else tells us to do so, but because we know personally, at the very center of our beings, what is right and what is wrong. Many years ago, Bishop Fulton Sheen expressed the idea in compelling terms: "Wrong is wrong, even if everybody is doing it, and right is right, even if nobody is doing it."

02 Winning: At What Price?

Do you want your children to be forced to become chemical stockpiles in order to be successful in sport, simply because of cheaters who are using drugs and who could not care less that they are compromising their whole sport?

There is nothing at all wrong with trying to win, unless you don't care how you win and what you have to do in order to win. Are you willing to cheat to win? Would you really think you'd won if you had to cheat to get there?

Cheating comes in many forms. Humans are nothing if not inventive when it comes to getting the "edge" in sport, as well as in other forms of human interaction. Even in social games like bridge, the adage "a peek is worth two finesses" is well known. In poker, cards have been marked and manipulated to increase the odds of winning. Auto racing is a constant exercise in breaking the rules without getting caught; tinkering with engines specs, hidden fuel tanks

CHAPTER TWO

and a variety of other efforts to circumvent the technical limitations. Hockey sticks have a specified maximum curve, but players are regularly caught with more than the allowed curvature. Baseball players are not above using corked bats, which are bats hollowed out and filled with cork to make them lighter and easier to swing. It was not long ago that major league slugger Sammy Sosa was caught with one and used the lame excuse that he had picked it up by mistake during the game and that he normally used it just for hitting exhibitions. This is the same home run king whom many believe is a doper, along with Mark McGwire and Barry Bonds. If so, perhaps being willing to cheat in one area inevitably leads to cheating in others. Every game and sport has its share of cheating.

Some cheating is just an ordinary attempt to get an edge over opponents, but some of it can be dangerous. High on the list of dangerous cheating is doping. Later, I describe some of the elements of the systematized doping programs of the former East Germany, not only on mature adults but also on young children who had no idea what was being done to them, in many cases until it was too late and there were permanent side effects. It does not take long before others recognize that some athletes are taking drugs and that they derive a performance-enhancing benefit from them.

If you are regularly getting beaten by someone who uses drugs, there are limited options available to you. You can report the use and face the consequences. Chances are that officials will do nothing about it, or worse, brand you as a whiner and try to marginalize you. You are unlikely to get much help from your fellow athletes, who may seem to have fallen into some kind of a code of silence on the whole question of doping. They know it is going on. They probably know who is doing it. They just don't want to talk about it. The cheaters will simply deny the use and continue to cheat.

Winning: At What Price?

Those with particular chutzpah and some resources will threaten to sue to frighten you, knowing that the defense of any action will be costly to you, no matter how little merit there is to their claim. Another option is to quit, but there is something particularly galling about being forced out of your sport because the cheaters have an insurmountable advantage. Or you can continue to get beaten and take whatever comfort you can from the knowledge that you are competing fairly and are losing to cheaters.

Yet another option is to try to beat them at their own game. Do the same things they do and level the playing field on your own. If you can beat them in a fair contest, chances are that if you take away their doping advantage, you can beat them again. If everybody is doing it, why shouldn't you? Maybe you won't get caught. Like all temptations, it is fairly easy to rationalize. And, almost before you know it, you become part of the same corrupt system—a drug user who professes clean sport in public and cheats in private.

One of the difficulties with this leveling of the playing field is that, once that particular "edge" disappears, the search for a new one begins. After all, the cheaters did not go through the exercise to achieve a level playing field. They did it to gain an advantage. If their advantage disappears, they'll want another one. If everyone is using two milligrams of a steroid, then maybe they will try four or eight. Do they care what the side effects will be? Maybe they will try substances that are far riskier, ones that have had little or no clinical research done to determine either the therapeutic or performance-enhancing characteristics. The search for the edge becomes addictive. And dangerous.

CHAPTER TWO

DO YOU KNOW YOUR KID'S COACH?

Let's face it. Coaches often have more influence on young people than their parents do. Do you have any idea whether your child's coach is someone who, as part of coaching, would be encouraging or condoning the use of drugs?

The primary relationship in sport is between the athlete and the coach. It is in the crucible of that relationship that great performances are born. Facilities, nutrition, funding and public support may be part of the overall picture, but they pale in comparison with the influence wielded by the coach, which is often more profound than that of parents. When I was an athlete, I had the benefit of superb coaches. Whatever I may have achieved was inseparable from their coaching and impossible without it.

It all started for me in a small pulp and paper town in northern British Columbia on the west coast of Canada. The town of Ocean Falls was built on the sides of two steep mountains separated by an inlet—on one side the mill, and on the other the company-owned town site for the approximately 3,000 people who lived in houses supplied by the company. The town was about 360 miles north of Vancouver, reachable only by boat or, for those with a death wish, by seaplane. Ocean Falls was an aptly named town, given its average annual rainfall of 230 inches. When we went to swim meets in Vancouver, the northwestern United States or in the Okanagan Valley, we were so pale from the lack of sun that I used to say we looked like fish bellies.

Because of the constant presence of water—whether the salt water inlet or the freshwater lake above the town—everyone knew how to swim. Sooner or later, you were bound to fall into one or the other. The company built an indoor pool, sixty feet long and twenty-five feet wide, and hired someone to look after it. It was heated, as was the whole of the town, by steam generated at the mill and piped to every house and building. The company, however, went one significant step further. The person hired to look after the pool and to give basic swimming lessons to the town folk was also a swimming coach. For almost my entire time in Ocean Falls, the coach was George Gate, who has gone on to be inducted into the International Swimming Hall of Fame and the Canadian Sports Hall of Fame.

I was lucky with my coaches, but many others were not. I know many who have had terrible experiences in sport as a result of bad coaching. I do not just mean coaches who did not know their profession well enough to create superb athletes, but rather those who could not motivate their athletes to do their best and to be positive about success, who were domineering, abusive, critical and negative. Nothing was ever good enough for them. Everything was measured in failures, and their athletes endured in a negative environment. They had to face the constant failure to meet expectations imposed on them by their coaches. They could never reach their full potential and could never enter competitions with the confidence that their preparations had been good enough to ensure that they would be successful. That kind of confidence makes the difference between winning and losing.

All coaches must know when to be firm, when to push, when to pull, when to be emotional and when to be thoughtful. They must know their athletes—what makes them tick and how best to get from them everything they are capable of achieving. They have to reinforce good habits, good results and successful teamwork, and persuade their athletes that even more improvement is possible if they work harder to achieve the goals they establish together. Not all athletes respond to the same approach, and what

CHAPTER TWO

separates the superior coaches from the ordinary or bad is the ability to tailor their approach so that each athlete receives the coaching he or she needs, in the manner that will maximize the chances for success and produce the best they are capable of doing.

I have always believed that parents should see their children's coaches at work. You do not want your kids in the thrall of someone who will encourage, condone or insist that they use performance-enhancing drugs. Some coaches believe that they are successful only if they produce "winners," and that their jobs are constantly on the line if they fail to do so. They have no commitment to the overall development of their athletes and no sense of how they will stifle and perhaps damage such development. Parents need to understand what the coaches are doing and how they are doing it.

After all, some coaches have seen their colleagues resorting to encouraging, even assisting, their athletes to use drugs. They all know, if they are paying any attention to what is going on around them, which coaches are involved in these practices. The results are normally all too apparent to be ignored. The drugs are taken because they work. The "clean" coaches will certainly be tempted to do the same. The key is to have coaches of sufficient character to resist that temptation.

Perhaps the best known doping scandal took place at the 1988 Seoul Olympics when Canadian sprinter Ben Johnson lost the Olympic gold medal in the 100 meters after he tested positive for the anabolic steroid stanozolol. His coach, Charlie Francis, understood that his athletes were competing with doped athletes. The evidence was all around him and he had no compunction whatsoever about doing whatever was necessary to compete against them. It was war. Their competitors used drugs, so his athletes also used drugs. He has always remained quite unapologetic about it, saying that drugs were part of the system and that there was no way his athletes were going to compete at a disadvantage, whether against the Soviet bloc athletes or those closer to home, especially when the system itself did not seem to care as much in practice about drug use as it did in theory. Charlie Francis is not the only coach on the face of the planet to have this attitude. We know about the East Germans and Soviet bloc coaches, some of the Chinese coaches and, in more recent times, Victor Conte and Remi Korchemny in the Balco scheme. There may yet be others identified in future as part of the continuing Balco fallout.

ARE PARENTS PART OF THE PROBLEM?

Do you know where the line is between support and encouragement, on the one hand, and pressure that might lead to doping? Are you trying to live vicariously through your child's success in sport? Are you in denial—or worse— about physical and emotional changes in your child?

The media are full of stories of fights, injuries and lawsuits surrounding sport, even children's sport. The scary thing is that many of the fights and injuries are not on the field of play, but in the stands, between parents or between the parents and the coaches. Some of these make road rage look like a pacifist convention. There's the father who filed his son's football helmet so that the opposing players were cut when hit by the helmet. And early in 2006 in France, Christoph Fauviau, the father of a tennis player, was sentenced to eight years in prison for having drugged his son's opponents to affect their performances. Unfortunately, as a result of the effects of the sedative, one of the opponents died in a car crash following a match.

CHAPTER TWO

I have seen parents hitting their children for failing to win a match, and coupling this physical abuse with verbal abuse that would make a sailor blush. What kind of message do they think they are sending? Children can learn as much from a bad example as a good one. We have all seen the parents who live their lives vicariously through the sporting success of their children, where the entire family effort is focused on the child and the athletic achievement to the point of obsession. Talent, ambition and focus can be good qualities; obsession is always unhealthy. Parents should follow through on their responsibility to ensure that their children are not ruined by sport and to retain some perspective on its relative importance in their lives.

There is also a great deal of "whistling past the graveyard." Many parents ignore obvious indications of drug use by their children. How many parents have said that they should have known something was going on—before there was a crisis? There is the sad case of seventeen-year-old Taylor Hooton who killed himself while in a depression resulting from steroid abuse. This tragic example received a great deal of sympathetic attention from the U.S. congressional committees during their 2005 hearings when his father, Donald, appeared to testify. There had been signs of a problem that had been ignored or dismissed until it was too late. If a child had an allergy or heart condition, you can be sure that parents would act immediately and without the slightest bit of shame. But, when a family problem involves drugs or alcohol or some form of mental illness, the shields come up and there is an astonishing ability to appear unaware of the problem. The fact of the matter is that these things do happen, not all with the same disastrous outcome, but nevertheless with serious and lasting consequences. Parents must be equally alert with their athletic children as with their couch potatoes.

THE WORST QUOTATION EVER

> *"Winning isn't the most important thing; it's the only thing."* It's the worst quotation ever. I wish Vince Lombardi had never said it. Winning is *not* the only thing.

It is all very well to say "Winning isn't the most important thing; it's the only thing" to a bunch of thirty-year-old professional football players. They can put it in context. But such is the immense influence of professional players and coaches that their sayings become watchwords for other athletes and coaches, no matter how far "off message" they may be for sport in general. Sure, everybody in competitive sport wants to win and will try their best to do so. But, winning is not the only thing. There is much more to sport than winning, and any coach who does not think so and says so to the athletes does not belong in the profession. The objective of good coaching should be directed at making the chances of winning better, developing the skills and building confidence.

It is not a failure to enter an event and not win, if the purpose is to gain experience for the future. I remember a swimming meet in Portland, Oregon, many years ago where I watched a younger swimmer try to complete 100 yards freestyle. He burst ahead, starting as fast as he could, setting a blistering pace. As it turned out, not only was he unable to maintain the pace, but he was unable even to finish the race. Was that a failure? Not unless he thought so. He was learning what he would have to do to be the world's fastest in that event some day. And, one day, he was the fastest in the world. Don Schollander won four gold medals at the 1964 Olympic Games in Tokyo. Some would have said that he "failed" in countless competitions before that, since, if winning each of those events was the "only" thing, all

CHAPTER TWO

his efforts had been wasted. I'm sure he smiles about that analysis when he occasionally takes his four Olympic gold medals out of the drawer.

This is, of course, an extreme example, and I chose it deliberately for that purpose. But the whole spectrum of performance and coaching is vitally important for sport. Any coach who thinks that winning is the only thing doesn't get it. I would not trust the judgment of any coach who thinks so. Nobody should.

I'll bet that there were days when Vince Lombardi himself had wished he hadn't made that much-quoted statement. He was, I am convinced, a better coach than that. I liked him better when he said, both about himself and his athletes, that if you were not fired with enthusiasm, you would be fired with enthusiasm.

Enthusiasm is the real point. The best people in every field are enthusiastic. We should be enthusiastic about participating in sport, about seeing how well we can do, about sharing the joy of effort and achievement, about having fun at the same time. Sport can teach us something about ourselves. Someone once remarked that sport does not build character, it reveals it. I think it does both.

If I were a parent who was thinking about what is best for my child, I would certainly encourage him or her to explore sport as one of the options. Physical activity is something that young people need in order to be healthy and alert. The social interaction, the fellowship, the sportsmanship that are inherent in sport are particularly valuable as part of their development and I can think of nothing better for them—unless it turns bad as a result of cheating or abusive behavior. If that happens, there are alternatives, whether music, the arts or some other form of self-expression, where many of the same disciplines apply, including teamwork, goal setting, working within defined criteria, measuring achievement and striving to be as good as possible. It would be a shame to give up the physical element inherent in sport, but that portion of the equation can be found outside the competitive sport structure that may have gone wrong. That is the risk that sport runs if the price of success is too high—people will vote with their feet and abandon sport. That would be a massive social failure and it would rest on the doorstep of those responsible for sport, who failed to deliver on the fundamental premise of sport: that it be fair.

SCANDALS

In this era of decline of ethical standards in business, the professions, politics, academia, the media and even organized religion, how could anyone expect that the same attitudes would not spread to sport as well?

Some day in the future, when there has been time for some perspective, historians may be able to tell us the reasons for the wave of misconduct at the end of the twentieth century and the beginning of the new millennium. Why was so little regard paid to ethics, whether in business, politics, academia, science, religion, the media or sports? Some of it will certainly be attributed to nothing more than greed. Some will undoubtedly relate to the lack of a strong moral basis for social conduct. But some may be far darker.

No one in our era can be unaware of the massive corporate scandals that have rocked the business world. All of us followed the fraud and corruption trials that included Enron, WorldCom, HealthSouth, Adelphia, Parmalat—the list goes on and on. Science is not immune from the same shortcomings. Pharmaceutical companies have been less than forthcoming about the risks associated with some of their products, even when their own data have shown that

CHAPTER TWO

such risks existed. The Merck Vioxx scandal of 2004 was just another in a series of pharma cover-ups. When such test data have not been disclosed or are otherwise discovered, the all-but-universal reaction of regulatory authorities tends to be a knee-jerk blanket withdrawal of the drug, even though there might well be some applications that are still worthwhile, even with better knowledge of possible side effects. In late 2005, a Korean genetic scientist announced that he had cloned a dog, but, not content with that, he went on to make a completely fraudulent claim to have perfected human cloning. It was regarded as a major breakthrough in the brave new world of genetic research, until he was forced to admit that it was all bogus. It was a shameful anticlimax and a warning that there are charlatans in every field.

Academia has its share of this type of conduct as well—both professors and students. Plagiarism is rife and cheating in examinations commonplace. Students hire writers for their term papers and other assignments. The publish-or-perish pressures of tenure-track academics result in publications that often have little or no academic merit. On behalf of the World Anti-Doping Agency, I recently wrote to the *International Journal of Sports Science & Coaching*, a supposedly peer-reviewed scientific journal that had published a 2006 article on doping in sport contributed by two academics that was so riddled with false statements, misinterpretations and unsupported conclusions that it was almost inconceivable that the article could have been published. I criticized the authors (to whom I wrote, without response, to ask if they planned to correct their errors), the so-called peer reviewers (who should, with even the slightest critical judgment, have spotted the errors and misstatements) and the editor (for allowing such rubbish to be published). The editor agreed to publish the letter.

Winning: At What Price?

The media are not exempt. In a business where being first with a story makes or breaks reputations, there has been a growing tendency to cut corners and to fail to verify information or, worse, to fabricate it. Even the mighty *New York Times* has been caught publishing stories that were frauds. Its internal controls were so lax that they did not pick up on major stories that were later revealed as complete fabrications. Dan Rather, the managing editor of *CBS Evening News* for over two decades, was forced into early retirement when he used false documentation as the basis for a national broadcast, ruining forever his reputation as a journalist.

Other journalists regularly make up facts and quotations or publish hearsay as fact, with no effort whatsoever to verify the accuracy of those facts. Opinion is often clothed as fact, and even in news stories, the public often receives not objective facts, but an interpretation of the facts, with no disclosure of the personal or institutional agenda of the reporter. And above all—here is some free advice that may be worth what you are paying for it—beware the journalistic "investigative" made-for-television shows, where the editors feel free to take whatever you say and use it to suit their own purposes, paying not the slightest heed to the context. I have participated in some of these and have personal experience on how a single sentence from a forty-five-minute interview may be inserted in the program to create a completely misleading impression of my views.

One major U.S. network, in my particular experience, was guilty of this. The network was CBS, and the program was *60 Minutes*. I had agreed to do an interview with CBS in Nagano, because they were the official broadcaster of the 1998 Olympic Winter Games, but Nagano was to be their last Games, so, as the IOC member responsible for television negotiations, I thought I should be cooperative. They did not say who the interview was for, and I thought it was for

CHAPTER TWO

CBS Sports. During the interview, the questions were very aggressive and non-linear. Someone from off camera and out of my sight would say things like, "ask him #17" or "ask him #23." Later, I found out it was *60 Minutes* and that it was essentially a hatchet job on the IOC president, Juan Antonio Samaranch. They had also interviewed him in English—not his native tongue—without disclosing the "investigative" nature of the program or that it would be about him in particular and highly critical. The network itself was so afraid of the *60 Minutes* editorial staff that, confronted with the obvious unfairness of the program prior to putting it on the air, it refused to do anything, even such as allowing Samaranch to answer the questions in Spanish. I have subsequently told CBS that I would be willing to come on to any live show and answer any questions its journalists may have, but I will never, ever, again be willing to be interviewed for their "investigative" cut-and-paste shows.

Revelations continue to surface regarding outrageous abuses within organized religion and its institutions. Innocent and needy people misplaced their trust in clergy, who were supposed to be spiritual advisors, and were systematically victimized by those whom they looked to for advice, guidance and comfort. Other church officials in a position to stop the abuse failed in their duty, at a terrible personal and emotional cost to the victims.

Do you see a pattern forming? Dishonesty, deviousness and duplicity—all leading to illegality, fraud and cheating.

Now, let's look at sport. I don't want to beat a dead horse, but sport is practiced within society, not in isolation. It is shaped and influenced by that society. It absorbs, inevitably, the values of the society within which it is practiced. But, and this is important, it also has its own values. The concepts of achievement, excellence, competition, self-discipline, teamwork and so forth are generally values that are reinforced by both sport and society. But when cheating in all other walks of life becomes commonplace, is it any wonder we see the same type of behavior in sport?

My point is this. Maybe the cheating in sport would have been publicly identified much sooner and been dealt with much more effectively if society as a whole practiced ethical conduct in so many other areas. Many have found it is simply better to close their eyes in this area as well, since it would not do for the pot to call the kettle black.

What price winning, indeed?

03 What Is Doping?

Doping can be dangerous to your health. How many parents of children who died from apparent heart attacks have made the connection between the loss of their loved ones and the drugs they had been using to improve their sport performances?

Imagine this scenario. John is seventeen. He plays on his high school football team. He's pretty good but is worried that he may not get into a good football college next year. His marks have not been as good as they used to be. He has become withdrawn and irritable when interacting with teachers, friends and family members. At home he sits in his bedroom, with the door locked. He doesn't even watch television much anymore. In the back of his closet is a bottle of capsules he got down at the gymnasium. The fellow who sold them to him said they would help him perform better and be stronger in his sport. He has used them now for a few months and there is no doubt that he feels stronger and

CHAPTER THREE

there are moments when he actually enjoys the practices and the games. But for every good moment, there are bouts of numbing fatigue, even though he knows he has no reason to be tired, and a feeling that everything seems to be going wrong. Maybe another of the pills will help, or perhaps two. There is a big game coming up, and there may be college scouts there to recruit from his high school. Possibly another pill the day before the game will help him to get noticed among the other players. If he can get an edge, it will all be worth it. Or will it?

One of the questions we often hear is "what is doping, and why all the fuss?" For one thing, doping can be dangerous to your health. Young athletes who take drugs are developing a whole range of symptoms depending on what they are using, whether it is as simple as severe acne or other, more worrying and potentially very dangerous effects. I describe many of these later in the list of substances and doping methods. Something that is often overlooked is the question of the long-term effects of doping. How will it affect the health of today's young athletes? There is a double problem here—most athletes never think anything bad will happen to them and, as for long-term effects, most athletes' horizons are such that they can barely conceive of the idea that, some day, they may actually be thirty, almost as old as their parents!

Unfortunately, it's too early to determine the final outcome, in particular cases, but the fact of the matter is that in addition to whatever sport doping athletes may be playing, they have also started a game of Russian roulette with their health. They may end up being lucky and not having serious side effects, but they may not. Ask the parents of athletes who have died from "heart attacks" in their twenties whether they think that drug use had some impact on what happened. Ask the current sufferers of heart,

What Is Doping?

liver, kidney and other disorders whether, if they could turn the clock back, they would still have used drugs to improve their sport performance. Ask the women in their twenties who are having trouble conceiving or whose children have fetal disorders what they think now about the drugs they took for sport, or the men who suffer from low sperm count and impotence if they still feel the invincibility of their youth. Would you give up the ability to have children for a momentary edge in some sport competition? Kids need to be protected from themselves if they do not have enough sense on their own. Parents, coaches and teachers, even friends, have to learn to watch for the signs. If drug use is stopped soon enough, many of the long-term effects may be eliminated or at least reduced.

Aside from the health issues, doping is cheating. It's as simple as that. It's breaking a rule that defines what sport is all about. There should be no place in sport for substances and methods that enhance performance, and if you resort to these, in the face of the agreed-upon rules, you are cheating and destroying an essential part of sport. It is just wrong.

Some people argue that drugs and other performance-enhancing methods are no different than diet, exercise and other physical training, which also enhance performance. They point out that modern equipment that enhances performance is not available to everyone, so why should anyone be concerned about unequal access to performance-enhancing drugs. Our society today uses pills and drugs for just about everything. So, why can't athletes use pills and drugs to improve athletic performance? But do we want a society that is over-medicated? Critics say that many anti-doping rules cannot be enforced because there are no tests for the newest designer drug. That, they say, makes sport a laughingstock—always behind, playing catch-up to the

CHAPTER THREE

cheaters. But constant progress in rule enforcement is being made by better tests and better testing programs.

Critics of anti-doping rules point out, in an obvious circular argument, that the use of drugs in sport would not be an infraction if there were no rules to prohibit their use. But sport cannot exist without rules. And that's the whole point. They *are* the agreed-upon rules. If the rules are no good, or even wrong, they may be changed. There are recognized and effective processes within the sport world to assess the rules and to change them if change is warranted. But, in the meantime, whatever the rules may be from time to time, they are the rules, and those who participate must follow them.

The doping rules were developed after many years of debate among those most connected with sport—the athletes, the sport officials and the public authorities of the countries in which the sports are practiced. The rules provide a framework in which sport can be practiced to the benefit of all concerned. Sport officials have concluded that doping harms athletes—physically, psychologically and socially. But while they all acknowledge that there should be rules against doping to protect minors, many of them, especially within professional sports, think that it's not necessary for adult athletes. What about the messages that superstar athletes send out? They have tremendous influence on impressionable young athletes, who conclude that what is "good" for star athletes—their heroes—must also be good for them. This is the message that is driven from the top down. Just what message did junior leaguers take away from the doping revelations about McGwire, Bonds, Canseco and scores of others? Even adult athletes may need protection from those who care little about their health, their bodies or their self-esteem, and who just want to use them to make money.

What Is Doping?

The people who endorse the rules (in particular, the anti-doping rules) have a positive view of what sport should be. They believe in the concept of the "spirit of sport," which is defined as "the celebration of the human spirit, body and mind." It is characterized by the following values adapted from the World Anti-Doping Code:

- ethics, fair play and honesty
- health
- excellence in performance
- character and education
- fun and joy
- teamwork
- dedication and commitment
- respect for rules and laws
- respect for self and other participants
- courage
- community and solidarity

This is what I think sport should be all about. It also reflects the combined views of the International Olympic Committee, all the Olympic international federations, all the other non-Olympic federations whose sports are not on the program of the Olympic Games, 202 national Olympic committees, the IOC Athletes Commission and 191 governments that adopted the 2005 UNESCO International Convention Against Doping in Sport. They have all chosen to embrace a vision of what sport should be and to adopt or approve rules designed to achieve that vision. Since doping is fundamentally contrary to the spirit of sport, they have identified a list of substances and methods (consistent with the World Anti-Doping Code) that should not be used in sport.

CHAPTER THREE

THE BANNED LIST

Nothing stands still. We have to do our best to keep up with the scientific developments used by cheaters. That means that the Banned List must be constantly reviewed and adjusted to be up to date.

Before WADA succeeded in establishing the World Anti-Doping Code in 2003, there was little international agreement on what substances should be banned. It seemed that each sport and each country had its own list. There was no continuity.

One of WADA's most important early successes in this area was to formulate a single "List"—the description of the substances and procedures that constitute doping. In doing so, WADA built on the IOC list, dating back to the late 1960s and expanded as the IOC learned of new drugs and procedures, that was used by many, although not all, international federations. This list is reviewed annually (or more often if there are special circumstances, such as the discovery that a new drug is being used for performance enhancement) by an international panel of scientific and medical experts. Substances or procedures are added to or removed from the list according to three factors:

1. scientific evidence that the substances or methods have the potential to enhance sport performance
2. scientific evidence that the use of the substances or methods represents a potential health risk to the athlete
3. use of the substance or method violates the spirit of sport

If two of the three factors are present, the substance or procedure may be added to the List. In addition, the List includes masking agents (which have the potential to hide or

What Is Doping?

mask the use of other prohibited things). Recently, finasteride has been used by many male athletes, they say to prevent hair loss. The problem with this supposed baldness paranoia is that finasteride is a recognized masking agent, so the drug has been added to the List for precisely that reason.

We have to do our best to keep up with the scientific developments used by cheaters, and that means that the List must be constantly reviewed and adjusted to be up to date. Each year, the proposed List for the following year is circulated to approximately 1,500 stakeholders (governments, international sport federations, national Olympic committees, athlete committees, laboratories, universities and other organizations with interests or experience in the field) for comments before it is finalized. With the exception of cricket, Australian Rules football and men's tennis, the professional sports leagues have studiously avoided any engagement with WADA regarding adoption of the Code. They do not want to have strict anti-doping rules and penalties. I deal with the professional sports in chapters 9 and 10.

Once the List is published, it is final for that particular year, and no one can challenge whether or not a particular drug or procedure should be on it. The List describes the substances and methods that are prohibited, and anything not on the List is permitted, even if it enhances performance. If something is not prohibited, there can be no penalty for using it. But one of the problems WADA has encountered is how to deal with all the possible variations of certain products, including those with trade names that vary from country to country. To avoid a List running to hundreds of pages, we use the scientific, pharmacological description of each. It's the responsibility of those using or administering substances to determine whether what they are prescribing falls within the description. The List includes substances and methods prohibited at all times (both in and out of competition) and others prohibited only during competition. Drugs prohibited at all times are listed below.

DRUGS PROHIBITED AT ALL TIMES

Anabolic Agents

Anabolic agents include those that may be produced by the body naturally as well as those that are produced artificially. Most of these are related to the male hormone testosterone. They can be taken orally, by injection and occasionally by application to the skin. Their properties are both anabolic (protein building) and androgenic (masculinizing) and vary by product as well as the body's own response. For the natural ones, a positive test occurs when the level differs drastically from what would be normal if produced naturally. Still, the athlete is allowed to try to prove that the level is due to a physiological or pathological condition. If combined with training, anabolic steroids increase muscle bulk, as well as speed up recovery times from training-related fatigue or injury.

Anabolic steroids have many side effects, some of which are reversible once you stop taking them. Others are permanent. Having effects similar to the naturally occurring hormone testosterone, they interfere with normal hormone function, leading to increased risk of liver disease, high blood pressure, increased risk of cardiovascular disease and even psychological dependence on the drug itself. In males, taking anabolic steroids produces acne, shrinking of the testicles, reduced sperm production, impotence, infertility, enlarged prostate gland, breast enlargement, premature baldness, potential for kidney and liver dysfunction and increased aggression and mood swings. In females, the effects include acne, development of male features, deepening of the voice, excessive hair growth on the face and body, abnormal menstrual cycles, enlarged clitoris, increased aggression and mood swings and fetal damage. If anabolic steroids are administered to adolescents, there will be severe acne on the face and body and stunted growth, in addition to the many other symptoms that will develop as they reach puberty.

Hormones

Hormones and related substances include erythropoietin (EPO), human growth hormone (hGH) and other growth factors, gonadotrophins (hCG), insulin and corticotrophins. They are normally taken by injection, although it is clear that some EPO applications are intravenous, since it appears that the detection period may be shorter if this method is used. Some of these hormones can be produced naturally, and there will be a positive test only when the level is outside normal parameters. But, as above, the athlete has the opportunity to prove that the concentrations are due to a physiological or pathological condition. If the test shows that the substance was not produced naturally, the test is positive.

EPO is a hormone produced by the kidneys that stimulates the production of red blood cells. Its synthetic version is used medically to treat patients with anemia associated with chronic kidney failure. The side effects include thickened blood, increased risks of blood clots, strokes and heart attacks, and risks of contracting infectious diseases such as hepatitis and HIV/AIDS if non-sterile injection techniques are used or contaminated needles are shared.

HGH is produced by the pituitary gland below the brain, which has the potential of stimulating muscle, bone and tissue growth as well as reducing fat. The side effects of HGH use include tremors; sweat; anxiety; diabetes in prone individuals; worsening of cardiovascular disease; muscle, joint and bone pain; hypertension; fluid retention; accelerated osteoarthritis;

acromegaly (distorted growth of internal organs, bones and facial features and the enlargement and thickening of fingers, toes, ears and skin) in adults; and gigantism (excessive growth of the skeleton) in young people. Human chorionic gonadotrophin (hCG) is a hormone produced by the placenta during pregnancy that can promote an increase in the production of natural male and female steroids. It can be found in small quantities in the urine of pregnant women. Because hCG stimulates the production of testosterone, the side effects can be similar to those experienced from anabolic steroid use, as well as headaches, irritability, depression, tiredness and rapid increase in height.

Insulin is a hormone produced by the pancreas and is involved in the regulation of one's blood sugar level. It acts on the metabolism of carbohydrates, fats and proteins. The side effects are severe and include low blood sugar (hypoglycaemia), which may then cause shaking, nausea, weakness, shortness of breath, drowsiness, coma, brain damage and death.

Corticotrophins are naturally occurring hormones produced by the pituitary gland to stimulate the secretion of corticosteroids. Use of these can lead to stomach irritation; ulcers; irritability; softening of the connective tissue; weakening of an injured area in muscles, bones, tendons or ligaments; osteoporosis; cataracts; water retention; high blood sugar (hyperglycaemia); and reduced resistance to infections.

Beta-2 Agonists
Beta-2 agonists, with certain limited exceptions for which a therapeutic use exemption (TUE) must be issued, are prohibited. These substances, many of which are used in the treatment of asthma, can enhance the flow of oxygen and, in the case of salbutamol, in sufficient quantities even have an effect similar to anabolic steroids. Side effects of use

include palpitations, headaches, nausea, sweating, muscle cramps and dizziness.

Agents with Anti-Oestrogenic Activity
These are normally used for treating breast cancers that depend on a supply of oestrogen for their growth. The side effects include hot flushes, weight gain, fluid retention, osteoporosis, thrombosis, ocular disorders, cardiovascular disorders such as venous thrombosis and hyperlipidemia, and liver toxicity.

Diuretics and Other Masking Agents
Diuretics are agents that help to eliminate fluid and minerals from the body by increasing the production or affecting the composition of urine. They stimulate the kidneys to increase the amount of urine produced to eliminate excess water and electrolytes from the body. Masking agents are products that have the potential to modify the excretion or concentration of other prohibited substances in urine, to conceal their presence in urine or other bodily specimens used in doping control or to change the haematological parameters. They too have side effects, such as fainting and dizziness, dehydration, muscle cramps, drop in blood pressure, loss of coordination and balance, confusion, mental changes or moodiness, and cardiac disorders.

Methods Enhancing Oxygen Transfer
Blood doping is a method that enhances oxygen transfer. It's the use of blood or red blood cell products of any origin or any artificial enhancement of the uptake, transport or delivery of oxygen.

Blood doping carries with it a number of obvious risks, such as allergic reactions ranging from rash or fever to kidney damage if the wrong blood type is used, increased risks of contracting infectious diseases such as hepatitis and HIV/AIDS, jaundice, circulation overload, blood clots, stroke or heart failure, and metabolic shock. Artificial oxygen carriers are chemicals used to increase the ability to carry extra oxygen in the blood. Side effects include a transient fever, reduction in the platelet count, potential overloading of the white blood cells, diarrhea, blood infections if the preparations are impure, high blood pressure, constriction of the blood vessels, kidney damage and iron overload.

Pharmacological, Chemical and Physical Manipulation

Pharmacological, chemical and physical manipulation of the urine is the use of substances or methods that alter or attempt to tamper with a sample. This can include covering up by using catheters, urine substitution and/or tampering, use of substances that modify or inhibit kidney excretion, and alteration of testosterone and epitestosterone concentration. There are infection risks with catheters, and the use of other substances prior to physical provision of the urine sample can have the side effects already identified.

Gene Doping

Gene doping—namely the non-therapeutic use of cells, genes, genetic elements or the modulation of gene expression—has the capacity to enhance athletic performance. Because most gene transfer technologies are still in the experimental phase, the full range of long-term effects of altering the body's genetic material is not yet known. But even from the early experiments, it is known that they can lead to the development of cancer, allergies and death.

What Is Doping?

DRUGS PROHIBITED DURING COMPETITION ONLY

Stimulants

Some stimulants—except those specifically listed as part of a monitoring program (to see how and whether they may be being used)—are prohibited outright, while for others there is a threshold below which a test will not be positive. Most are taken orally. Because many of these can be generally available, often without prescriptions, the List is drafted to provide some flexibility that allows lesser sanctions to be imposed where it can be shown that there was no real attempt to dope. Side effects of stimulant use can include serious cardiovascular and psychological problems, such as overheating of the body, dry mouth, increased and irregular heart rate, increased blood pressure, increased risk of stroke, cardiac arrhythmia and heart attack, visual disorders, problems with coordination and balance, anxiety and aggression, insomnia, tremors, dehydration and weight loss.

Narcotics

The use of narcotics—including heroin, methadone and morphine—to reduce or eliminate pain can be dangerous, since the substance merely hides the pain and does nothing about the cause. Some are taken orally, some injected and some can be inhaled through smoking. Pain is often nature's way of telling you that something is wrong. Continuing an activity because it no longer hurts may lead to further and possibly permanent damage. Other dangerous side effects include slowed breathing rate, decreased heart rate, sleepiness, loss of balance, coordination and concentration, nausea, vomiting and constipation. We have also seen feelings of euphoria, invincibility and illusions of physical prowess beyond the person's actual ability, which may put the person and those around him or her at risk. Prolonged use can lead to physical and psychological dependence, and eventual addiction. Excessive use can suppress the respiratory system and be fatal. Many of them are also illegal, the possession or use of which may lead to criminal prosecution.

Cannabinoids
Cannabinoids—such as hash and marijuana—have psychotropic properties, which in small amounts can cause a feeling of relaxation, reduce inhibitions and pain and can cause a loss of perception of time and space. They are usually smoked, but may be eaten as well. Because they may alter perception faculties, they could put the safety of both the user and persons around him or her at risk. Other effects may include a state of drunkenness, drowsiness and hallucinations; reduced vigilance, balance and coordination; reduced ability to perform complex tasks; loss of concentration; increased heart rate; increased appetite; and mood instability (rapid changes from euphoria to depression). Even for marijuana (regarded by some as the least offensive of the cannabinoids), long-term use may lead to loss of attention and motivation, impaired memory and motivation, weakening of the immune system and respiratory diseases such as lung and throat cancer and chronic bronchitis. While I find it hard to imagine that they are likely to be performance enhancing, there are some who believe they are and who insist that they be considered accordingly. The U.S. authorities consider marijuana to be the entry-level drug for more pernicious drugs that have greater effects on users.

Glucocorticosteroids
When administered orally, rectally, intravenously or intramuscularly, use of glucocorticosteroids requires a TUE. Topical

What Is Doping?

preparations—when used for dermatological, nasal, buccal cavity and ophthalmologic disorders—are not prohibited and do not require TUEs.

These are substances produced by the adrenal gland that are able to regulate numerous functions in the body, particularly inflammation. When administered systemically into the blood, glucocorticosteroids can produce a feeling of euphoria. Corticosteroids, the most powerful anti-inflammatory agents available in medicine, are used in the treatment of numerous non-infectious diseases that are characterized by pathologically inappropriate immune or inflammatory reactions. They also relieve pain and are commonly used to treat asthma, hay fever, tissue inflammation and rheumatoid arthritis. When administered into the blood stream, glucocorticosteroids can have numerous side effects, such as osteoporosis; fluid retention; softening of connective tissues; weakening of injured areas in muscle, bone, tendon or ligament; increased susceptibility to infection; heartburn, regurgitation and gastric ulcers; alteration of blood vessel walls, which could result in the formation of blood clots; disorders of the nervous system, such as convulsions and muscle cramps; psychiatric disorders, such as changes in moods and insomnia; and decreasing or stopping of growth in young people.

Other Drugs

There are certain other substances that particular sports prohibit in competition, such as alcohol and beta-blockers. Alcohol can relax the athlete and reduce basic tremors that may affect aim and coordination, but may also create a danger to other competitors, as might be the case in power boating or automobile or motorcycle racing. Specified thresholds vary from sport to sport. For competitors in shooting, beta-blockers are also prohibited at all times.

CHAPTER THREE

Specified Substances

"Specified substances" are particularly susceptible to unintentional anti-doping rule violations because of their general availability in medicinal products or because they are less likely to be successfully abused as doping agents. Where there is a doping violation involving a specified substance, there is the possibility of a reduced sanction, provided that the athlete can prove that the use of the substance was not intended to enhance sport performance. These include inhaled beta-2 agonists, probenicid, ephedrine, cannabinoids, alcohol, glucocorticosteroids and beta-blockers.

That will give you some idea of what is "out there" when athletes participate in sport and the lengths to which many are willing to play—or allow others to play—with their bodies, body chemistry and manipulation of bodily functions and blood. The humanism of sport risks being overtaken by the pharmacist, leaving the athlete reduced to little more than a laboratory experiment, with the next new and improved body just around the next test tube.

04
Test Tube Athletes

What if there were something that would enable you to train harder, with less rest and less fatigue than other athletes? Something to give you the edge. Wouldn't that be tempting?

Training for competitive sport is hard work, especially when there is aerobic demand and strength involved. Perfecting skills is equally difficult at times, but often not as debilitating as trying to build up endurance and strength. When you are training, you are always tired and often hurt. A million years ago when I was a swimmer and going far less distance than the obscene yardages imposed on today's athletes, my constant feeling was one of exhaustion and wishing I could have a day off. When there were two training sessions a day, I sometimes felt like a sleepwalker, dragging myself to classes at university. God knows what the professors thought of the yawning student in front of them.

CHAPTER FOUR

Now, leaving aside the ritual complaining about the hard work that is common to all athletes, success involves training—plain and simple. The training, in addition to improving your performance, demonstrates to you that, yes, you can perform perfectly well, even though you think you can barely move. And, yes, I did develop a resting pulse in the mid-thirties, so there was considerable progress in the ability of my body to handle the stress of high performance. Also, it is fundamental to the whole nature of competitive sport that you have to be able to produce when you are under stress. The only way you can learn to do this is to create conditions of stress during training so that you will know what it feels like and so that your stroke or stride or swing will not break down as quickly when you are getting to the limits of your capacity. You know from your experience that you can endure a bit more (you hope) than the other competitors and you live for the sight of your opponent starting to fall slightly behind or your closing of a gap that may have been opened early in a race.

But, what if there were something that would enable you to train harder, with less rest, less fatigue than other athletes? What if the build-up and accumulation of lactic acid could be drastically reduced, if muscle tears induced by training were miraculously cured? What if more oxygen could be delivered to your muscles than you have been able to generate through the months or years of training? What if that something came in a bottle, a pill, an injection? What if only you knew about it and your competitors did not?

EAST IS EAST

> *East German athletes were given doses of "vitamins" as part of the training regime. To remain part of the team, they had to follow the instructions and take the vitamins. They did not ask any questions.*

Test Tube Athletes

When you think about drugs and sports, one of the first things that springs to mind is the former East Germany. The German Democratic Republic was the unacknowledged master of systematic doping in international sports. Following the post-war division of Europe, the country was completely dominated by the Soviet Union. It had virtually no independence, and the only area in which it felt it could shine was sports. In a totalitarian state, if those in power want a sport program, a sport program is what they get.

It was not until 1972 that the IOC allowed East Germany to field its own team at the Olympic Games. Munich's Olympics was really the first time that the world saw what remarkable progress the East Germans had made in sport. They came in third in total medals, ahead of West Germany and behind the USSR and the United States. By the time of the Montreal Games four years later, the East Germans moved up to second place, ahead of the United States. They were no longer merely remarkable; they had become dominant, so much so that it was becoming generally known, although it could not be proven at that time, that there was chemical enhancement involved. Manfred Ewald, the East German sports minister, was the mastermind of the country's remarkable success. He had not the slightest compunction about using any means to give his athletes a competitive edge, including drug programs. In fact, he organized the design of the programs.

If you were an East German athlete, you were given doses of "vitamins" as part of the training regime. The athletes were told that if they were to remain part of the team, they had to follow the instructions and take the vitamins. They did not ask any questions, despite the noticeable side effects. Women's shapes and sizes changed. Their voices grew deeper, they developed acne, changes occurred in their genitalia and they were subject to mood swings. What mattered to the central planners, however, was that they also got better, stronger and faster. By the time of the Montreal Games in 1976, the question in women's swimming was not how many gold medals the East Germans would win, but whether anyone else could win any.

One of the finest of their swimmers was Kornelia Ender, an attractive but very large young woman. How big? I could stand behind her and you could not see me. Her calves looked bigger than my thighs. She dominated the freestyle events. Some of her teammates looked like they had been sculpted out of rock, so pronounced was their muscle definition. Swimmers from other countries looked like frail little girls compared to these East German warriors.

And, make no mistake about it—the Manfred Ewalds of the world viewed them as cold warriors. They were at the Olympics to demonstrate the superiority of their political system. They were servants of the state, with no other purpose. They had been identified and trained at the expense of the state and with all of the resources of the state, and they were expected to perform accordingly. And they were expendable warriors.

AND WEST IS WEST

> *Although everyone denied it, we were doping, too—not with the same systemic rigidity of the Soviet system, but in a typically entrepreneurial Western way, in a free-enterprise society.*

It would be wrong to think that this sort of thing was going on only in East Germany and the Soviet bloc. There were many in the west who saw sports through the same lenses as their Cold War opponents. Sport was a way to demonstrate the inherent superiority of a political system or philosophy.

Victory on the playing field was just as satisfying as military victory, but much less expensive, and the politicians did not have to deal with explaining daily body counts to the media. Medal counts and world records were examined with minute attention.

We were all too eager to point fingers at the Soviets and the East Germans and cry doping, but when it came to our side, improved performances were all said to have resulted from better training methods, equipment and facilities, sports psychology and so on. These did play a role, but a glance at the results leads us to conclude that they were *too* good. There was another factor that no one was talking about—doping. Even at that time, doping was forbidden in sports. How, then, do you go about discussing the unmentionable? The easiest solution seemed to be to deny the existence of any problem. There were no drugs in sport. Drug use simply did not happen. Not with us—we were the good guys.

This was nonsense. We were doping, too—not with the kind of structured programs applied across the whole spectrum of sport that marked the central planning popular within the Soviet bloc, but in a typically unconnected entrepreneurial Western manner, in a free-enterprise society. Instead of a system, there were pockets of initiatives, in which the doping was done entirely within the private sector. Both sides worked in secret, however, because everyone knew that using the drugs was against the sport rules to which they both publicly, loudly and sanctimoniously subscribed. America's medal winners were its heroes, and they had to be sure that their feet of clay did not show. So, drug use developed, and a code of silence built up around it.

CHAPTER FOUR

GUINEA PIGS

> *Who knows how many of the heart attack deaths of young athletes have resulted from the use of performance-enhancing drugs and the resultant stress on a heart that has to pump blood with the consistency of sludge? At the very least, it is reckless experimentation with the athletes as subjects. At worst, it could be criminal.*

Take the recent case of Kelli White, a talented American female sprinter, who won the 100 and 200 meters at the 2003 Athletics World Championships in Paris. Her tests were positive for a stimulant called modafinil. Normally, this would have led to her disqualification, but her entourage produced a certificate from a doctor who said he had been treating White for narcolepsy and had prescribed this psycho-stimulant "as required" to keep her from suddenly falling asleep. Her handlers claimed that this was a medical condition and not an example of doping.

At the time, I remember hearing that explanation and was amazed that anyone could possibly think it would fly. Modafinil was something that needed to be taken regularly by a narcolepsy sufferer. You do not take it *after* falling asleep at the wheel while driving your car on the highway. Was there some danger that she might fall asleep in the starting blocks or during the eleven or so seconds of the 100-meter race? The suggestion was incredible. Finally, White's handlers argued that modafinil was not really a stimulant, and that therefore the positive test reported by the laboratory was meaningless.

The International Association of Athletics Federations (IAAF), which is the governing body for athletics (track and field), did not buy the argument. There had been no application by the athlete for a therapeutic use exemption

(TUE), which enables athletes with genuine medical conditions to apply for permission to use certain prohibited substances in the treatment of a condition. TUEs are granted (or refused) by a committee of experts, and they have to be satisfied that a genuine medical condition exists and that there are no viable alternatives to the prohibited substance for treatment of the condition. And, particularly important, the TUE must be applied for prior to the event, not after the fact, when urine samples show positive drug results, as was the case with White.

The IAAF also disputed the suggestion that modafinil was not a stimulant. Because there was a lot of prize money at stake and because athletes ritually deny any drug use, even in the face of obvious evidence to the contrary, the matter was appealed to the Court of Arbitration for Sport. White was found guilty, and her medals and prize money from the event were withdrawn.

OK, that all seems perfectly normal. Someone used a stimulant and had not filed a TUE in time, which might have avoided the whole problem. Sadly, there was much more to all this than originally met the eye. Around the time of the World Championships in Paris in 2003, the Balco scandal was beginning to break, and with it came revelations of the names of athletes who had been clients of Balco. One of the clients was White. A major product distributed by Balco was the designer steroid THG. From the records of the Balco files, it turned out that modafinil was not White's only drug use. She was also a user of THG. Unlike some of the athletes in the Balco thrall who persisted in their denials, once this information came to light, White agreed to accept a two-year sanction and to assist in the prosecution of other cases with which she was familiar, and to speak out against doping in general. Several cases are pending, while others have been decided.

CHAPTER FOUR

It gets worse. White accepted an invitation from the World Anti-Doping Agency to appear at our meeting in Montreal in May 2005. There is always some risk in agreeing to such appearances, since there might be different agendas being pursued, such as arguments in favor of allowing athletes to take whatever they want and for the "old guys" to butt out. Instead, as a result of her appearance, our board members were able to get a first hand inside view of some pretty seamy practices in U.S. athletics.

According to White, her story, in some respects, was quite simple. She had started to run at the age of ten and continued at university, hoping it would one day become her career. After university, she reconnected with her former coach, Remi Korchemny, one of the central figures in the Balco affair. Shortly thereafter, in 2000, Korchemny introduced White to Victor Conte. Korchemny said that she just needed some nutritional supplements, proteins, vitamins and energy drinks, which she took. Korchemny told her that one of the products was flaxseed oil, but she learned afterward that it was, in fact, THG.

In 2001, she decided to stop using all the products, but then had a series of injuries and was not enjoying any success. She and Korchemny decided to go back to Conte, and the "cocktail" settled upon consisted of THG (taken by needleless syringe under the tongue), EPO (injected once a week around her stomach), a masking agent in the form of a cream rubbed on the inside of her elbows and a mixture of stimulants to take prior to the start of races. The treatment started in March 2003 and continued for at least four months. The results were unbelievable. She doubled her workload in training, developed significantly more muscle mass and ended up on top in the world championships in Paris that August, before the modafinil-related disqualification. By the following May, she had acknowledged the Balco and THG elements of her program.

Why was she doping? She was not blind. She saw the results that Korchemny had achieved with other athletes under his wing, including Michelle Collins, who has since been sanctioned as well. That success was influential in making the decision to go ahead with the Balco doping program. She knew she would have to change something in her preparation in order to get to the top. As far as her coach was concerned, it was completely ridiculous for her not to do so, and he told her that she did not have the natural talent, without doping, to ever make it to the top. Since the Balco revelations, White said she had had nothing to do with Korchemny, who she considered to be, on a technical basis, a good coach. Not without some misgivings, she did as he suggested, thinking that he had her best interests at heart. She began using THG. She was told that it was undetectable and that she should not worry about being caught.

She was more worried about some of the physical side effects, including the fact that she was having menstrual cycles every two weeks. So Conte and Korchemny reduced the dosage. It was clear, if only in retrospect, that they had no idea what the side effects would be and that they were experimenting on White. She was nothing more than a guinea pig for them. She developed severe acne on her face and chest, and her voice was transformed significantly. Probably the most dangerous side effect was a serious rise in blood pressure, which took a long time afterwards to get back under control and within a normal range. Korchemny's only response was to tell her to drink more water. And so it went.

She had seventeen doping control tests prior to the world championship, both in and out of competition—all negative, because, unlike today, there was no test for THG at the time, since only a handful of users knew it existed.

CHAPTER FOUR

And, as to EPO testing, they all knew that it was performed only on runners going 400 meters and farther. The popular belief at the time was that EPO did not provide sprinters with any advantage, so the testers did not bother to test the sprinters. The stimulants also seemed to have gone undetected. How, she was not sure.

Coming up to the 2003 World Championships, the Balco crew was still not worried about the possible detection of THG. The only question was whether they should up the ante by providing White with the modafinil, which they thought should be OK, since it was not specifically listed as a stimulant by name. (The list does not give the name or trade name of every drug, or it would be too voluminous. The main stimulants are listed, and the others are included under the general language.) They decided to take the chance, and that was what led to White's original downfall. Conte had said that he was 110 percent certain that it could not be detected by the IAAF and was not on its list of prohibited substances. White did not think she needed it to win, but took it anyway, just to be sure to win the races.

It was Dr. Brian Goldman, apparently a "consultant" for Balco, whose certificate, presumably an after-the-fact TUE, was provided to the IAAF. He said he had met White on three or four occasions and had prescribed the modafinil for the narcoleptic condition from which she had allegedly suffered. White says she had never met this doctor and had never had any narcoleptic condition. She had never heard the word "narcolepsy" before it was trotted out as a defense against the positive test.

Here was a doctor Conte apparently had in his stable who was willing to lie, professionally, as part of a scheme to help athletes cheat, so don't be fooled by all of the protestations of innocence you may hear. Just like others who cheat, Kelli White was quite willing to play out the charade until the Balco revelations made it impossible.

White's view was that if WADA wanted to be effective in the fight against doping in sport, we would have to increase the angles of attack. This meant focusing on athletes, coaches and better investigation of the distribution of the drugs being used. There were other athletes ready to speak out and there were still, even with the demise of Balco, lots of things going on "out there." Some athletes were continuing to ask how to get hold of the doping products. The coaches were the key, since they were the ones advising the athletes. Everyone knew who the bad ones were. As for White, she wanted to get back to athletics, maybe to become world class again, and she was filled with remorse for what she had done. Oddly enough, at the time, she was quite happy about winning the 100 meters, but, as for the 200 meters, she was disturbed, since she had won too easily and by too great a margin, which was not normal.

White speculated that money was a motivating factor for doping athletes, since many athletes are consumed by the desire to have money. She had started to win some money herself, was running only on good tracks and in good meets, had a reserved warm-up facility and traveled in luxury conditions. When you win, you are well treated. You travel in limos. When you are not at that level and you see the difference with your own eyes, you want the same things. And you convince yourself that you are not doing anything wrong. At the time White spoke with us, Korchemny was not only still denying any responsibility in respect to the Balco indictments, but was still coaching athletes. On April 19, 2006, White announced that she would not be coming back to competition.

That is the type of organized conspiracy that faces athletes who would like to compete drug-free. Dopers are

CHAPTER FOUR

well funded, interconnected, ruthless and unapologetic, capable of denying flagrant abuse with a straight face and no apparent conscience that they have cheated. They do it over and over again and will continue to do so until they are caught. Even then, they take advantage of every possible technical defense their lawyers can dream up. What's more pathetic is that such nonsense occasionally works.

What happened to the East Germans and to Kelli White is by no means limited to them or to their countries, or even to their sports. It has certainly happened in my country, and we enjoyed, for a few years following the Ben Johnson incident at the 1988 Seoul Olympics, considerable notoriety when he was stripped of his gold medal in the 100 meters. Since that time, Canada has endeavored to combat the problem more aggressively and has become known as a country with a fairly vigorous anti-doping policy. On the other hand, we have not completely eradicated the practice. Nor has any country. Nor has any sport, despite what they may say.

Certain countries are farther behind than others. There is still a less-than-adequate degree of transparency in many of the former Soviet republics and access to them for independent testing remains a challenge. The same is true of China, and many are concerned that the run up to the 2008 Olympics puts Chinese athletes at even greater risk, especially when it has been revealed that some of the leading coaches working in China today were former East German coaches. There had been several cases in the late 1990s of doped Chinese athletes, especially in swimming, making astonishing and remarkable progress in that sport, as well as the finding of doping substances in their possession during the world swimming championships in Perth, Australia, in 1998. The Chinese seem to have taken this to heart and there has been a combination of no further positive tests and a significant diminution in the performance of their swimmers. India has had a rash of positive tests and has been slow to react to an evident problem, but, as the hosts of the 2010 Commonwealth Games, they will be required to respond with more enthusiasm and effectiveness than they have shown to date.

The real problem is that no one is able to monitor what is going on at the level of the individual gymnasiums or sports clubs, where the drugs are distributed and the temptations begin. There is probably a parallel between the initiation to performance-enhancing drugs and the social drugs, possibly with the try-the-first-one-free approach, plus the "Everybody's doing it, why not you?" Or, "If you want to be any good you have to do the drugs—don't be a fool." It is pretty insidious. One of my children attended a fine college in New England. He was on the swim team. Someone asked him if he wanted to make some money selling dietary supplements to members of the team. There was nothing illegal, he was assured—just nutritional supplements. He asked me what I thought, and this was long before I had become involved in WADA. I said that he should stay away from the whole thing, especially since no one could ever be sure what the supplements contained. The labeling regulations in many countries—including the U.S.—are so weak that the producers could put almost anything in the supplements and have no responsibility. But an athlete who had taken a tainted supplement could test positive and face a penalty. My son would not want to be involved in anything that could jeopardize his teammates, not to mention create legal problems for himself.

It's hard for me to say this, because the coaches I had were such extraordinary influences on my life that I wish that what now happens with too many of them were not true. But I think that coaches often vary between not

CHAPTER FOUR

wanting to know about drug use and actively encouraging it. They get paid on the basis of results and if their results are not good, they may be unemployed in short order. So, maybe they abandon part of their moral responsibility in the process. I insist that no coach worthy of the description can be unaware of drug use by someone in his or her charge. It is, for example, no accident that the tip-off on THG came from a coach. Coaches know what is going on in the field and who is doing it. It was one of the straight-from-the-heart statements that Charlie Francis, Ben Johnson's coach, made when he said that doping was the norm and that if his athletes did not use the drugs, they would be at a competitive disadvantage. They work on technique, equipment, facilities, so why not on their bodies? Why not chemically?

All over the world, there are people with similar attitudes who have enormous influence over young athletes. The values they teach are often tragically wrong for everything sport should represent.

TEST TUBE SUCCESS

Is this sort of thing happening to your kids? Are they someone's test tube experiment or guinea pig? Do you know where your children are?

Drug-taking athletes and their entourages do not want to share their advantage with others. They want it for themselves, for the edge they hope it will give them in a competition. If everyone had the same stuff, the relative advantage would be canceled out and everyone would be back where they started. And, sooner or later, everyone *will* get the same stuff. Now what? Now there is a search for something new, or perhaps a higher dosage. What if, instead of two pills per day, you take four? Maybe the effect will be twice as good and you will regain the advantage.

In many cases, the drugs being used are already dangerous to one's health. When you get to the next level of abuse, the risks increase exponentially. No one has any idea what the impact will be. The designer steroid THG, which was given to Kelli White, was strong enough to double the frequency of her menstrual cycle. It was easy for those giving the stuff to her. After all, it was not their bodies that had to absorb and deal with the THG. Who knows what this may have done to her reproductive abilities, to her heart, her liver or to other vital organs? Who knows how many of the heart attack deaths of young athletes, particularly in cycling, have resulted from the use of EPO and the resultant stress on a heart that has to pump blood that has thickened to the consistency of sludge? At the very least, it is reckless experimentation with the athletes as subjects. At worst, it could be criminal. Is this sort of thing happening to your kids? Are they someone's test tube experiment or guinea pig? Do you know where your children are?

05
Doping Is Not an Accident

Understand this—doping in sport is almost never, I repeat, almost never accidental. It is almost always planned and deliberate. It is carried out with the specific intention of enhancing performance, knowing that it goes against the rules of sport and that it is dangerous to the health of the athlete.

I should make something clear at the outset: doping is not accidental. OK, maybe, once in a while, the occasional athlete may take a cold tablet by mistake or ingest tainted nutritional supplements without the slightest intention of doping, but, believe me, these cases are very few and far between. Taking anabolic steroids is not accidental. Seeking out, paying for and using THG and other "designer" drugs at $3,000 a pop is not accidental. Paying $40,000 per year for the supplies and treatments exposed in Spain just prior to the 2006 Tour de France is not accidental. Taking EPO is not accidental. Blood transfusions and manipulations are

CHAPTER FIVE

not accidental. Genetic doping, when it becomes a reality, will not be accidental. Inserting a device in your anus filled with "clean" urine to avoid providing your own sample is not accidental. This last form of cheating has become so common that the rules now require that athletes providing urine samples must be bare from thigh to chest so that doping control officers can observe how the urine sample is provided. That is how the IOC caught a Hungarian discus thrower, at the Athens Olympics. Female athletes also catheterize clean urine directly into the bladder, through the vagina. In early 2006, an Indian weightlifter was found with a container of "clean" urine strapped to his waist. Artificial penises, known as whizzinators, can be purchased over the Internet. They have only one purpose—to beat doping tests. Onterrio Smith, a running back with the Minnesota Vikings, was stopped in April 2005 in the Minneapolis-St. Paul International Airport in possession of an "Original Whizzinator." It was not for purposes of impressing his girlfriend; it was specifically designed and used for the purpose of avoiding a positive drug test. The Canadian Football League has become a summer camp for NFL players serving out their suspensions. Both Smith and Ricky Williams have been welcomed with open arms to the CFL. I have seen some of these devices. They are disgusting. The people who make them are disgusting. The athletes who use them as part of their cheating, and those who assist them in such efforts, are disgusting.

Systematic doping is generally associated with the east bloc countries that had been doing it since the seventies, but many other nations are also guilty. In Atlanta in 1996, we learned that for several years, Soviet athletes had been treated with, among other things, a stimulant called bromantan. The IOC tested an athlete, found it and declared the athlete positive, but the Court of Arbitration for Sport overturned the disqualification on the basis that bromantan had not been specifically mentioned as a stimulant. That disappointing decision allowed several other Russian athletes in Atlanta to escape without penalty. We know the network of western coaches and athletes that enabled cheaters such as Ben Johnson to reach the heights of his performance. We have seen the cycling teams that systematically used doping products for their riders. We saw the sudden, extraordinary performance improvements among Chinese athletes, some of whom were linked to coaches from the former East Germany. We have seen reports of entire soccer teams being doped. The same seems to have been true for at least one of the NFL teams—the Carolina Panthers. These are not accidents. They are organized programs.

The reports of systematic doping in cycling make it clear that there is a doping industry in play. Whether or not the teams themselves are organizing the doping, there can be little doubt that it has become a very serious problem for the sport. There are known medical doctors and scientists regularly sought out by riders. The Spanish revelations in mid-2006 show how deeply the doping culture is embedded in cycling, but there are athletes from other sports involved as well, including track and field. In cycling, it is also clear that the suspected riders are not just the ones at the back of the peloton, but those at the front, the pretenders to the position of Lance Armstrong, with the extraordinary record of seven straight wins in the Tour de France. Many of them were withdrawn by their teams on the eve of the 2006 Tour, following their identification in the Spanish investigation. Cross-country skiing and biathlon are also rife with doping and have had to increase their testing programs.

One of the techniques that had to be put in play—I hope only on an interim basis—is the so-called health test. If a blood sample shows that the red blood cell level

CHAPTER FIVE

(known as the hematocrit level) is beyond an established "normal" range (which is far beyond normal for you or me), that might indicate doping. To simplify things and speed matters up, when abnormal red blood cell levels are found, authorities do not bother trying to prove that doping has occurred. They simply refuse to let the athlete participate, saying (and not without reason) that it would be unhealthy for the athlete to do so. Few athletes protest, perhaps because many of them are happy not to have been formally caught.

This process does two things. First, it identifies cases where there is a genuine risk to the athlete. Second, it is a fast and easy way to get a cheater out of the event. In the case of cycling, the quarantine period is fifteen days, while for the winter events, the athlete is allowed to start once the hematocrit level falls below the established threshold, which could take two to three days or longer. Athletes often argue that the level is normal for the person, or that the higher altitude increased the level. While training at high altitudes does result in more red blood cells, these protests often ring hollow, given the extraordinary levels achieved and the coincidence of having such levels on the eve of a competition. I even heard of one athlete who ascribed the high hematocrit level to the fact that he had taken a flight and that the lower oxygen levels due to the cabin pressure had stimulated his red cell production. Who do they think they are fooling? As an instant solution for a particular event, the health test is fine. A potential cheater has been removed and will not taint the competition. Half a loaf is better than nothing at all. What should happen thereafter is that the athlete be marked for targeted testing on a regular basis, to determine whether doping is occurring, and that longitudinal records be kept of the athlete, so that the results of tests can be compared with previous results and variations noted that might indicate doping.

Doping Is Not an Accident

In Turin, a couple of days before the 2006 Winter Olympics, there were a dozen or more cases of abnormally high hematocrit reported from the limited number of samples taken by the International Ski Federation (FIS). Was this doping or mere coincidence? As a practical matter, the athletes were kept from participating until their levels got back to normal. In the future, I hope all the athletes involved will be identified for target testing. For WADA, it was too convenient a coincidence—so many high levels, so close to the Games—so we decided that we should organize a session with international experts on blood doping.

Meeting after the Games, the experts agreed that some of the cases were probably due to doping. The hematocrit test alone was not enough to confirm an official doping offence for EPO, which requires urinalysis, so there was no way to impose sanctions. The meeting underlined the need to quickly develop tests for EPO and related compounds. At present, tests must be administered within a couple of days of EPO usage because it disappears from the system. It leaves a high level of hematocrit but that is not enough to convict, hence the need for out-of-competition testing. At the meeting, it was also decided to compile historical data on each athlete as part of a longitudinal follow-up, so that significant changes could be used as an indication of doping. If the cheaters are going to be systematic, why should we not be systematic as well?

REPEAT OFFENDERS: AUSTRIAN HIGH JINKS AT TURIN

Did this signal the end of the age of innocence of the Olympic Games? Were athletes to be regarded as potential criminals? Were they forever tarred as a result?

CHAPTER FIVE

Some people never seem to learn, even when their schemes are exposed. Following the Olympic Winter Games in Salt Lake City in 2002, cleaning personnel in rented quarters used by the Austrian cross-country skiing team outside the Olympic Village discovered a raft of materials—vials, needles and similar stuff—that could have been used for blood doping. The Austrians were called upon to explain. They insisted that this paraphernalia was not used for blood doping, but to keep their athletes from catching colds! Apparently this was done by transfusing their blood, irradiating it with ultra violet rays and then retransfusing it back into the athletes. This explanation, unsurprisingly, did not impress anyone. The coach of the athletes, Walter Mayer, was fired by the Austrrian ski federation but later reinstated. He was banned by the IOC from any Olympic Games until at least 2010 and by the FIS from any skiing competitions for eight years. The Austrian decision was appealed and was unresolved at the time of the 2006 Games. Maybe there is no domestic Austrian interest in resolving it. None of the athletes who may have used the process were disciplined, because they did not test positive before or during the Games.

There were elements of a James Bond intrigue surrounding the same team in connection with the Winter Games in Turin in 2006. As part of the anti-doping program relating to the Games, WADA agreed to cooperate with the IOC and the various international sports federations to conduct unannounced out-of-competition tests in the lead-up to the Games. No one thought the Austrian cross-country and biathlon problem had simply disappeared. The FIS had the Austrian federation in its sights and WADA had also followed the events from Salt Lake City. So, it was no surprise when WADA's doping control officers were requested to conduct some no-notice tests on Austrian cross-country skiers and biathletes during their training periods. When the doping control officers arrived at the Austrian hostel, operated by Mayer and his wife, where the athletes were supposed to be staying, they were unable to locate any of the athletes or their coach; however, they did find equipment and supplies that could be used for blood doping—containers, needles and blood testing or manipulation devices, including a centrifuge.

Unfortunately, doping control officers are not authorized to seize property, even when it is clear that it has been used for doping activities. But their suspicions were clearly aroused and when they submitted their report of the missed tests to WADA—if an athlete is not where he or she is supposed to be when a doping control officer arrives to collect a sample, it counts as a missed test—they described what they had found. We filed the information away for future use. The next step in the drama occurred shortly before the Games when WADA doping control officers were collecting samples from a number of teams in the Turin region. They came upon a photograph of the Austrian cross country team and there, lo and behold, was the smiling photograph of Mayer as the coach. Our doping control officers casually asked a number of people in the area if they had seen Mayer. Several had and pointed out the place he had rented. The doping control officers advised WADA accordingly.

I thought we should advise the IOC of this suspicious collection of facts. It may all have been entirely innocent, but given the experience at the previous Games, the absence of the athletes, the finding of the equipment, the presence of Mayer in separate premises outside the Olympic Village and his position as coach, we felt that the IOC should know what we had found and what the implications might be. The IOC agreed and also thought that the Italian authorities should be advised, since some of the possible activities were contrary to Italian law.

CHAPTER FIVE

Working together, the IOC and the Italian police decided to conduct their respective tests and investigations at the same time. On the evening before one of the races (the time when top-up blood doping is most likely to occur), the police and testers entered the premises occupied by Mayer and noted that the athletes present, who were requested to provide urine samples, began to drink enormous quantities of water, obviously trying to dilute their urine so that it would be difficult or even impossible to detect the presence of EPO. Someone threw a bag of supplies out the window, hoping that the bag would get up and run away, perhaps. The Italian authorities seized the bag as evidence. It is not clear whether the combined operation was leaked, but a few of the Austrian athletes had already left the country, apparently worried that they could be tested. WADA was sent to find the athletes in Austria and to test them, which we did, but by that time there was nothing to be found.

The Mayer part of the story becomes rather odd at this point, because he left Italy shortly after and then engaged in some inexplicable conduct. There were suggestions in the media that he might have been contemplating suicide. In any event, a police pursuit in Austria ended with Mayer crashing his car into a police barricade. He was taken to hospital for treatment and psychiatric evaluation. Mayer seemed to have been concerned whether he could justify his presence in Italy solely as a spectator. This was, as might be expected, a big story in the media.

This time, the matter did not stay under the scope of the Austrian radar. The Austrian Chancellor, Wolfgang Schüssel, visited IOC President Jacques Rogge during the Games, initially to complain about the treatment of the Austrian athletes. But when given the underlying facts (apparently his staff had not fully briefed him), his position changed to publicly questioning how it was possible for a person like

Mayer to have been involved with Austrian athletes. Mayer was again dismissed from his position. Opposition parties called for anti-doping legislation and, not unpredictably, criticized the government for its *laissez-faire* attitude. The Austrian Olympic Committee took its skiing federation to task and launched its own inquiry into the matter. The IOC established a disciplinary committee to look into the facts. New Austrian legislation was enacted.

The public prosecutors in Italy began to realize the implications of what they had found when they searched the premises occupied by Mayer and some of the athletes—including supplies and equipment that could be used for blood transfusions. Two of the Austrian athletes, by now back in Austria, announced that they were retiring from competition. Mayer, upon his release from psychiatric observation, apparently filed criminal complaints in the Austrian courts against Rogge and me, allegedly for criminal libel. I say "apparently" since I have only read this in the media and have not been served with any official or court documents. I called Jacques Rogge to see if we could perhaps arrange to share a jail cell in Austria. He, too, had not been served with any official court documents. Rumor also has it that Mayer is considering suing WADA itself for entering the hostel where the doping control officers, looking for the athletes who were supposed to have been there, had first observed the supplies. So far he seems to have spared the Chancellor from any legal action. Oh, yes, and—surprise, surprise—the Austrian ski federation solemnly cleared Mayer of any involvement in doping.

Both media and athletes questioned whether the actions of the IOC and the police were appropriate in the circumstances, or extreme. It was definitely the first time that such combined actions were taken by the IOC and police during an Olympic Games, at least in the matter of doping.

CHAPTER FIVE

Did this, in some way, signal the end of the age of innocence of the Games? Were athletes to be regarded as potential criminals? Were they forever tarred as a result? Was this a situation that could only arise in Italy because it had enacted a special law dealing with the use of drugs in sport?

The situation in Italy is unusual because Italy is one of very few countries that has penal sanctions regarding drug use contained in a statute that is specifically sports-related. It is more unusual because most countries have stayed away from penal laws that are particular to sport. That does not mean, however, that in other countries it would be impossible to apply penal sanctions to athletes and others in relation to the possession, supply, trafficking or use of drugs such as anabolic steroids. Almost all countries have general laws of this nature, that do not necessarily focus on sport but, on the other hand, could certainly be used in relation to sport. In the United States, for example, steroids are controlled substances that cannot be used without a prescription and I believe (just ask Victor Conte) that possession as well as trafficking are criminal offenses.

The practical answer, therefore, is that most countries probably do not need a specific statute dealing with drugs in sports, as is the case with Italy where there is a sport-specific law, to get to the same bottom line. It requires only a new or additional focus on enforcement of the existing legal framework, if there is a will to have governments get tougher on doping within sport. The legal means to prosecute offences within sport already exist without the necessity of a special sport statute. In fact, I doubt, for example, that the U.S. or Canada would even consider the enactment of a specific statute dealing with drugs in sport and that much the same view would exist in the vast majority of western countries. It would take very little to imagine the police and the IOC working together in similar circumstances in the next Olympic Winter Games in Vancouver in 2010, without needing the muscle of new legislation. Not only has the combined action in Turin been an operational success, but it sends a message to potential doping cheaters and their entourages that there is now a new level of cooperation between the sport and public authorities, the latter using the powers they already possess, whether under specific sport legislation or the general criminal law system. This should have a significant impact as a deterrent, especially for those who provide the drugs or other assistance for doping. It is just one more example of getting at the suppliers as well as the users.

In the meantime, the Italian authorities are examining the evidence that they collected at Mayer's quarters outside the Olympic Village and will decide whether they have sufficient grounds for laying penal doping charges against Mayer and any athletes who may have doped. The Austrian Olympic Committee has launched its own investigation, and WADA has provided the Italian and Austrian investigators with copies of the reports it gave to the IOC. The IOC has begun an investigation and is currently waiting for the outcome of the Italian authorities' procedures before reaching its own conclusions. A full description of what had been seized by the authorities may go a long way toward establishing precisely what the Austrians may have had in mind, especially if the seized materials happen to include containers of blood. Even possession of a prohibited substance by an athlete can be a doping violation, unless the athlete has a properly granted TUE or other acceptable justification. It is not necessary that there be a positive test result before a doping offence can be said to have occurred. If the supplies and equipment are consistent with doping, then there will have to be a very good explanation for their presence if those involved are to escape without a doping sanction.

CHAPTER FIVE

In one sense, it is not the end of the age of innocence of the Games. As far as doping is concerned, that already happened decades ago when organized doping began to occur. What has changed is that the IOC is simply more determined than ever to ensure that the Games are more innocent—in the sense of being doping-free—than ever before and that it is prepared to use all available means, including close cooperation with the public authorities, to do so.

No one regards all athletes as potential criminals, but we do insist that they follow the rules and that they be prepared to prove that they comply. That is a sport rule, not one falling under the criminal law. In some countries there may also be criminal laws, and if you happen to be in one of them, it is up to you to make sure you don't run afoul of the law. Are you forever tarred as a result of being caught as a cheater? Probably. And so you should be, even after you have served your sanction and have been allowed to come back. I have always liked this statement attributed to President John F. Kennedy: "Forgive your enemies. Never forget their names."

I repeat—doping is very, very seldom accidental. It is almost always planned and deliberate. It may be sophisticated, such as blood manipulation, or it may be as simple as a standard stimulant or anabolic steroid, but it is not an accident. If you think it is, I have a bridge in Brooklyn that I would like to sell to you.

06
Testing: Games People Play

I have often thought about the idea of sponsoring a contest for the most original excuses for testing positive for dope. But who could we get to judge these creative liars? And what criteria could we use?

Many athletes live a lie, and I suppose you have to expect it. Athletes use drugs, and they lie about it. Even when they get caught, they lie about it, with denials and excuses that defy the imagination. One of my favorites is, "I have never knowingly taken drugs." This was an amusing fallback for Rafael Palmeiro, baseball star with the Baltimore Orioles. He was so adamant that he had never taken drugs that he swore to this fact under oath in congressional testimony, punctuating the fact with a pointed finger. Within months, he tested positive for steroids and was suspended for ten games, and his previously unshakable, unequivocal, rock-solid position was watered down to the thin and unconvincing gruel of never "knowingly" using drugs.

CHAPTER SIX

What, did somebody spike his Gatorade? I don't think so! It was so ludicrous that the congressional committee seriously considered prosecuting him for perjury. They eventually decided that there wasn't enough evidence to convict him but that did not mean he hadn't lied. It was a case of "not proven" rather than "not guilty."

DOPING EXCUSES

The truth of the matter is that once banned substances are found in an athlete's system, there is no excuse. It doesn't matter how they got there.

Here are just a few creative doping excuses that I have heard over the years.

- Rafael Palmeiro said that his positive test for steroids must have resulted from some tainted vitamin B_{12} given to him by a friend.
- Javier Sotomayor, the Cuban high jumper who tested positive for cocaine, claimed it was a CIA plot.
- Dennis Mitchell, a U.S. track and field sprinter, said his positive test for a testosterone-based drug was the result of having had sex four times the night before and drinking six beers. He should at least be convicted of being a braggart!
- Dieter Baumann, a German runner, after testing positive for nandrolone, claimed that his toothpaste had been spiked.
- In Australia, cricketer Shane Warne said his mother had given him a diuretic so that he would look slimmer on television, without mentioning the shoulder injury from which he was trying to recover. The diuretic was a masking agent that could have hidden the possible use of steroids

that would help the injury cure faster. He had returned to play almost twice as quickly as the experts had predicted.

- In a similar vein at the Australian Olympics, kayaker Nathan Baggaley said that he unknowingly drank some steroid-spiked orange juice in the family fridge. It was there because his brother, also an athlete, was using the drink to recover from an injury. Some healthy family fridge! A Court of Arbitration for Sport (CAS) arbitrator ruled, how I can-not imagine, that there were extenuating circumstances—no "significant fault"—and reduced the normal two-year suspension to fifteen months. Now the sport authorities are investigating the brother!
- In Argentina, tennis player Mariano Puerta said he accidentally used some of his wife's menstrual pain medication, which led to his own positive test.
- U.S. cyclist Tyler Hamilton said the reason why his blood test showed two types of blood in his system, indicating that he had blood from another person in him, was that he must have had a "vanishing twin" who disappeared during his mother's pregnancy, but whose blood was nevertheless still there and part of his own. After sticking with this absurd story through a complete arbitration process where the argument was rejected, Hamilton eventually abandoned it in his subsequent appeal, which also failed, and was convicted of blood doping.
- Austrian cross-country ski officials said that the blood transfusion equipment found in their premises in Salt Lake City following the Winter Games in 2002 had been used to treat the skiers to avoid colds. The excuse was that replacing their blood would keep them from getting colds or would cure them.

CHAPTER SIX

- Barry Bonds said that as far as he knew, he was just taking flaxseed oil and that was what accounted for his unexplained growth spurt so late in life.
- NHL goalie José Théodore said he was using finasteride, a masking agent, to fight against hair loss.
- Sesil Karatantcheva, a sixteen-year-old Bulgarian tennis player who tested positive twice for a steroid called nandrolone, said she did so because she had been pregnant in May 2005 at the French Open, but the tests performed at that time did not confirm this. She then said that she had had a miscarriage.
- Several tennis players suggested that their positive tests for nandrolone might have resulted from tablets provided to them by officials of the Association of Tennis Players (ATP), the organization that runs men's professional tennis. They did not provide the slightest proof that there was any connection whatsoever. This gave the ATP a convenient excuse not to sanction the players because, though far-fetched, had the unsupported suggestion been true it would have been the ATP's fault that the players had taken the drug. The ATP could not possibly penalize the players for something the ATP itself was responsible for. Only former Canadian and current Briton Greg Rusedski was identified as one of the tennis players in question. The identity of the others, perhaps some of the "stars," has been kept carefully hidden by the ATP.
- A U.S. skeleton athlete, Zack Lund, tested positive for a masking agent. He blamed it on his use of finasteride, a hair replacement drug that he had been using for some time, although it had never showed up in previous tests analyzed in the U.S. Very curious. He was exonerated by the U.S. Anti-Doping Agency, but WADA appealed against that exoneration to CAS and he was suspended for having used a masking agent.

Testing: Games People Play

- Two Kyrgyz athletes, skater Anzhelika Gavrilova and biathlete Jamilya Turarbek, were banned prior to the Turin Olympics for positive tests of clenbuterol, a substance used to promote muscle growth, and furosemide, a masking agent. Turarbek said that she took the diuretic to help her urinate. Really!
- C.J. Hunter, a U.S. shotputter, who tested positive for steroids at least four times in 2000 leading up to the Sydney Olympics, claimed he took a tainted iron supplement.
- Lithuanian cyclist Raimondas Rumsas claimed that the thirty-seven different doping substances seized in his wife's automobile were for his mother-in-law.
- Latvian rower Andris Reinholds claimed he took a Chinese herbal remedy—made in the United States.
- Belgian cyclist Frank Vandenbroucke said the EPO that was found in his possession was for his sick dog.
- Chinese track coach Ma Junren said his athletes were only eating dried caterpillars and turtle soup.
- Uzbekistan athletics coach Sergei Voynov, who was caught smuggling fifteen vials of human growth hormone through the Sydney airport prior to the 2000 Olympics, said the drugs were to treat his baldness.
- French rugby player Pieter de Villiers tested positive for ecstasy and cocaine and claimed that possibly his beer had been spiked.
- British athlete Paul Edwards tested positive for a combination of anabolic steroids and clenbuterol, and claimed they must have been in some shampoo he had drunk!
- Japanese billiard player Junsuke Inoue claimed the presence of the anabolic steroid methytestosterone in his system was not designed to enhance his performance in billiards, but in the bedroom.

These are just some of the wild excuses used by athletes who tested positive for dope. Stay tuned. There will undoubtedly be further and greater stretches to our imagination coming along in the future.

Of course, in the long run, it does not matter (nor should it) how or why the substances were ingested, since the rules make the athletes responsible for whatever may be in their blood streams. Once the banned substance is found in their system or there is an attempt to use a prohibited method, the doping offence is complete. The circumstances are relevant only in assessing the penalties that should apply, as in the cases of Baggaley and Lund, noted above. But this has nothing at all to do with the question of whether or not there has been doping.

THE "I HAVE NEVER TESTED POSITIVE" MYTH EXPLODED

> *"I never tested positive" is a mantra. For sophisticated cheaters, it means nothing more than they've never been caught, especially when they know there is no test for what they've been taking or doing. It is not "proof" that they have not doped.*

It is always interesting to see the fallback positions of athletes who are suspected or accused of doping. There are several mantras that come into play. "I have never tested positive" has become so commonplace that it is a wonder anyone was ever fooled by it. This statement is trotted out as proof that the athletes in question have not doped—no positive result means no doping. End of any possible controversy, they say. But, the statement is true only as far as its contents take it. The only thing it proves is exactly what it says—that the person has never tested positive. It doesn't prove whether or not the person has used the prohibited substances or methods. It simply means that they never got caught if they were doping. Often, it was because there was no test at the time for the substance they were using.

There are many ways to beat the tests. For many years, cheaters smuggled in clean urine, hidden on their person or in bladders concealed in body cavities, which they provided instead of their own. That is one of the reasons why doping control officers are required to observe that the sample is provided properly. Other means included timing of the use of the drugs so that the athletes' systems would have "cleared" by the time of the tests, while still retaining the performance-enhancing benefits. Some drugs clear within a matter of days. Others use masking agents that disguise the prohibited drugs. There are no reliable tests yet for certain substances, like human growth hormone, that enable testers to go back several weeks or months. Even though hGH can be detected, the body produces it naturally in some quantities, and so far it has not been possible to easily differentiate the natural from the added hormone on a basis that will satisfy the scientists (but we're working on it). In sports like cycling, where athletes selected for testing have no chaperone for up to an hour before they present themselves for testing, or where they are tested several hours before their races, instead of immediately before they start, there are opportunities for manipulation, such as catheterization or dilution. Cheaters and their entourages are nothing if not inventive.

The Balco debacle showed the importance of having tests for the latest drugs. THG was being used on a regular basis. The athletes were tested but because there was no test for THG they did not test positive, despite the fact that their systems were chock full of it. In fact, they were encouraged to use the stuff because Conte assured them it would not be

CHAPTER SIX

detectable. So, with the appearance of wide-eyed innocence and barely suppressed moral indignation of even being suspected of organized cheating, they pointed to the results of the repeated tests and declared proudly that they never tested positive. As a combination of hypocrisy and affrontery, it is hard to beat. How many athletes have been denied their wins by these cheaters? How many athletes who competed fairly had to stay home and watch the Olympics on television while the doped-up athletes who beat them in the trials by cheating competed in their place, proudly representing their countries? How many non-doping athletes in other sports were beat out by dopers?

Most of the Balco athletes (other than the professional players, so carefully coddled by their leagues and players' associations) have either finally admitted that they cheated with the help of Conte, Korchemny and others, or have been found guilty by arbitration panels. Some have admitted that they used TGH, while others were found guilty, in most cases, with precious little difficulty. The headline "I have never tested positive" will forever be associated with the case of Tim Montgomery, a former world record holder in the 100 meters and former partner of Marion Jones. Montgomery had never tested positive, a fact that he used repeatedly as the answer to all his accusers. But, it was all too clear from the many records seized from Balco and the testimony given by Conte to the prosecuting officials that Montgomery was a client of Conte and a user of THG.

This led the United States Anti-Doping Agency (USADA) to declare in June 2004 that Montgomery had committed a doping offence. This triggered the usual flood of denials as well as an appeal. Under the international rules governing track and field, the first level of appeal is to the national authority, in this case a USADA appeals board. Then, if the outcome at the national level is unsatisfactory for either party, or if the international federation decides that the rules were improperly applied, the matter goes to the international level. Montgomery chose to short-circuit the procedure and appeal directly to the Court of Arbitration for Sport (CAS), which is the final authority in all matters of doping, bypassing the initial level of appeal in the United States.

Since Montgomery did not test positive, there was no doubt that it was up to the USADA to prove that a doping offence had occurred. The USADA presented mounds of evidence, including documents from the Balco investigation and Montgomery's blood and urine test results. But it was the testimony of Kelli White, the track and field athlete who had earlier admitted to doping with Balco assistance, that had the biggest impact. She testified that Montgomery had admitted to her that he used THG. Ouch. That must have hurt! It was now up to Montgomery to refute that evidence, but he didn't. His lawyers called no other witnesses, and Montgomery himself did not even give evidence. He even refused to refute the damning evidence given by White, even though the CAS panel bent over backwards to give him a chance to do so.

Based mainly on White's evidence, the CAS concluded that Montgomery was guilty of doping. This case was a significant step forward and has put a stake through the heart of the "I have never tested positive" argument—that the only way to get a conviction for doping was by obtaining a positive blood or urine sample. The panel pointed out that there were several ways to demonstrate that a doping offence had occurred other than positive dope test results.

This opens up the possibility of convicting dopers who use substances or doping methods that we cannot detect with the available tests. For example, a commercial test kit for the use of human growth hormone (hGH) is still being developed. There are athletes out there who have been

CHAPTER SIX

using hGH believing that they will not get caught by a test. They probably are saying, "I have never tested positive." Imagine if Victor Conte is willing to give evidence to a CAS panel that what he said on the ABC network television program *20/20* in the spring of 2005 was true—that he sat beside Marion Jones, dialed up a shot of human growth hormone and watched her inject it. That could be sufficient to establish a case of doping. What if the CAS panel accepts that evidence, the way the Montgomery panel accepted White's evidence? The same could be true for blood doping and other substances for which there are no current tests.

There are some who wonder whether all this might be going a bit too far. Should there not be a requirement to have a smoking gun, in the form of some positive doping test, before an athlete can be punished? The answer is no, because other evidence is just as valid as a positive test. All the more so if there is not yet a reliable test for the substance or method that may be being used. Other evidence that can lead to a conviction includes confessions by the doper, evidence of eyewitnesses and consistent circumstantial evidence.

The Montgomery case was a real breakthrough in the fight against doping in sport. Evidence other than a positive dope test could be used to determine guilt or innocence. Now that even the possession of prohibited substances without a TUE, trafficking and attempts to use such substances can be a doping offence under the World Anti-Doping Code, the net has been cast much wider than ever before. Those who are aware of doping or who see it attempted or who know that athletes or coaches have prohibited substances in their possession can now do their part in exposing the cheating, based on the Montgomery precedent. The gloves are off.

So, dopers beware! You now have an additional risk of not knowing if and when someone will come forward and expose you as the cheaters that you are. Montgomery was convicted. He was guilty. Oh yeah, and he had never tested positive.

07 Why Do We Need to Regulate Doping?

After the Tour de France scandal in 1998, with half the Festina team in police custody for suspected doping, cycling in disarray, the IOC under suspicion as soft on drug use and other sports perceived as equally uncommitted to the fight against doping in sport, a new dynamic was required. Nobody believed anybody anymore. And with good reason.

The World Anti-Doping Agency, WADA, was founded partly as the result of the doping scandal during the 1998 Tour de France, when the French police found industrial quantities of doping substances on one of the teams. IOC President Juan Antonio Samaranch was not deeply committed to the issue. To him, the fight against doping was more of a nuisance than a gut issue. He made all the customary anti-doping statements, although he was not ready to rock the doping boat, creating tensions between the IOC and the international federations, who did not want any outside interference in their affairs.

CHAPTER SEVEN

But he did, inadvertently. As Tour de France's Festina team athletes and officials were being arrested for possession of the doping supplies and equipment, Samaranch blurted out that, for him, this was not doping and that the IOC's list of prohibited substances and methods was too long. He felt that a substance should be banned only if proven damaging to health. He had forgotten that a journalist was present. The next day, the story came out that the IOC president disagreed with the anti-doping policy of his own organization, a policy that he himself had repeatedly supported in public. It was a very explosive story and gained momentum in the media. The IOC was castigated for its now-revealed hypocrisy regarding drugs in sport. No one was willing to believe the IOC was serious; similarly, no one trusted the international federations to police activities in their own sports, and no one believed national authorities would be as hard on their own nationals as they would be on foreigners.

It was the French police, not the cycling organizations—whether the Tour de France officials, the Union Cycliste Internationale (UCI) or the French cycling federation—who uncovered the doping and had taken action. It was no different in other sports. It was embarrassing for international federation officials to acknowledge that their sport was infiltrated by cheaters, so they didn't. At the national level, when was the last time you heard of a positive test by China, Bulgaria or Romania on one of its own athletes? Countries regularly covered up or minimized tests they performed on their athletes. If the dopers are caught and exposed, it is by other testing agencies; they don't call fouls on themselves. The Greek athletics federation refused to find Kenteris and Thanou guilty for missing tests prior to the Athens Games in 2004. Elaborate hoaxes were created in Athens to provide excuses and explanations. Genuine enforcement only happens if there is an independent anti-doping organization, and there were all too few of them in existence. It was, in short, a mess, and in 1998, a very public mess. As a result, the process of establishing WADA began.

BIRTH OF WADA

> *The situation was a complete mishmash. Each sport had its own rules—or didn't. Each country had its own rules—or didn't. The confusion led to a public perception that no one was serious about doping. Something had to be done. Only a completely independent international agency could provide the necessary credibility—WADA.*

We needed to try to restore some sense of integrity in the fight against doping in sport. It was, by now, all too clear that the process could not be controlled by the IOC, since it had been exposed by its president as less than fully committed. My suggestion was that it would require an entirely independent agency and one that no stakeholder was in a position to control. The structure we settled on was one that involved both the sport movement and governments. While sport often resents government involvement in its operations, this was an area in which we needed their help and they had also been quite critical of the efforts from within the sport movement to get a handle on the problem, especially, although unfairly, the efforts of the IOC. To move things forward, the IOC organized a world conference on doping in sport in early 1999, with the hope that the conclusion would support the establishment of the independent agency. Things got very sticky when governments insisted on a 50-50 governance structure, but it turned out to be a blessing in disguise for the sports movement, for two reasons. First, it meant that we would

CHAPTER SEVEN

not have to fund the entire cost of the agency by ourselves. Any stakeholder that wanted half the control could hardly justify not paying half the costs. Secondly, it meant that governments would now have to become proactive in the fight against doping in sport, especially after their harsh criticism of the sports movement. Once the principle of the agency was approved at the conference, the next step was to negotiate the governance mechanics and get it into existence, which we managed in record time. WADA was created in November 1999 and began its operations in early 2000. The voting members consisted of an equal number of representative from the Olympic Movement and of the governments from all five continents. We did not make an initial approach to the professional leagues because the crisis affected mainly the Olympic sports and the IOC and we knew that it would only further complicate an already complex set of relationships to add them to the mix. Besides, we had no programs in place that might have some application to them. That would come later, when the World Anti-Doping Code was adopted.

I can assure you that I had no idea that I would end up being involved in its operations, much less being its president. With great initial reluctance, both because of the additional workload and because I had never had any connection with anti-doping activities, I agreed to take on this role, but only for a couple of years, until it was up and running. It didn't work out like that—I'm still there, despite the prolix efforts of Lance Armstrong to have me removed.

Two early objectives of WADA (which were met in the first year) were: 1) to be in the field, doing out-of-competition tests in the lead-up to the Sydney Games, and 2) to have an independent observer checking the doping control process at the Games. Once the agency was established, it became apparent quite early on that one of the greatest

Why Do We Need to Regulate Doping?

difficulties in the fight against doping in sport was the huge variations between the rules in different sports and different countries—and the level of their enforcement.

There was a confusing quiltwork of rules, with different sanctions, different procedures, different lists and different testing protocols. In some sports, like rowing, the rule was a lifetime ban from competition for the first offense. In others, a first offense might be no more than a private warning not to do it again and no one else would even be aware that a doping infraction had occurred. In some sports, once there was a positive dope test and the doping review process had been completed, there was an announcement of the infraction and the penalty, while others maintained confidentiality even after the sanctions and the affected athletes faded away, just like old generals. Some sports did not recognize sanctions imposed by other sports, so that you might be suspended from competition for doping in cross-country skiing, but still be able to compete in athletics or cycling. Cheating was not transferable.

There was never any way to determine whether adverse laboratory results had been acted upon and confirmed (or not) as cases of doping. There is a distinction between an adverse analytical result reported by a laboratory and a positive doping case. The laboratory result may show, for example, the presence of a particular drug in the system of the athlete, but there may have been a valid TUE that allowed the athlete to use that particular drug. Other times the quantity of the drug may have been less than the threshold provided for a positive doping case. That had happened when British sprinter Linford Christie had tested positive during the 100 meters at the Seoul Olympics in 1988, but the quantity was small enough that the IOC Medical Commission ruled, by the slimmest of majorities, that it was not taken for purposes of doping.

CHAPTER SEVEN

It was all the more goofy because when the British heard the rumors of an important athlete in the 100 meters having tested positive—who later turned out to be Ben Johnson—they called a press conference to confess that it had been Christie!

Developing countries had far more important priorities than regulating sport. International federations could not control their national federations, so different rules, and different sanctions in case of positive tests, applied in the same sport, depending on where a test was conducted or a game was played. Some national federations simply refused to follow the rules established by the international federations and would not comply with requests for information on doping cases. Most notable among these examples was USA Track & Field (USATF), which stonewalled the IAAF for years, refusing requests to provide information concerning at least thirteen U.S. athletes guilty of doping offences but "cleared" by USATF in secret proceedings.

Some federations had rules, but no means of enforcing them and no processes to test the athletes and discipline them when doping was discovered. National Olympic committees in each country grouped all their national federations under one roof and tried to manage the different rules that each member federation applied. Athletes were confused as to which rules were in force when and where, and what substances and methods they were allowed to use and which were prohibited. Coaches and advisors had the same problems. Officials charged with enforcing the rules seldom knew where to turn. The confusion led to a public perception that no one was serious about doping, despite what they might say in public. Something had to be done.

Why Do We Need to Regulate Doping?

BIRTH OF THE WORLD ANTI-DOPING CODE

> *It was little short of a miracle that the WADA Code came together so quickly. But WADA's adoption of the code was only the beginning. The code meant nothing until the sports movement and governments acted to incorporate it into their own rules.*

We decided that the ideal solution would be to organize and harmonize the rules, so that the same rules would apply to all sports, to all athletes and in all countries. The question was how to get from the existing chaos to the result we hoped to achieve—the creation of a single World Anti-Doping Code. There was not much difficulty in getting support in principle for the idea from most of the stakeholders, including the governments, though they knew how complicated the project would be. The IOC was also supportive, having tried for some time, with little success, to have its own single code. The athlete members were keen but had no idea of how a single code could be achieved. The key was to attract the interest of the international federations (IFs) and to engage them in a collaborative exercise that would not compromise their authority to govern their sports, but would improve the efficacy of the fight against doping. We did some informal sounding out of the idea with a few IFs that had considerable experience in the field and were assured of their cooperation if we decided to proceed. And proceed we did.

As the first official draft that would be circulated took shape, the working group expanded its circle of consultation, to get more input and to broaden the range of consensus. After several months, they were ready to send out a first draft of a proposed code to every conceivable stakeholder, including governments, IFs, national Olympic committees

CHAPTER SEVEN

(NOCs), athlete groups, laboratories, professional associations, leagues, international agencies, medical doctors, experienced sports lawyers—anyone we could think of that might have some interest in the subject matter of the proposed code. Although it was the first draft unveiled, so to speak, in public, I think it was our sixteenth or seventeenth draft. The process was repeated three times, so that no one could legitimately say there had been no consultation. We set an end date for the process and settled on calling a second World Conference on Doping in Sport in early March 2003, approximately four years after the first world conference in Lausanne in 1999 that had led to the creation of WADA. Copenhagen was selected as the host city.

I won't go into the dynamics of the Conference, other than to say that after three days of tough sledding, we had unanimous approval of the sports organizations and governments present that the draft Code was acceptable, so the WADA Foundation Board adjourned to formally adopt the Code and returned to report that the Code was now in existence.

At the Copenhagen conference, the eighty governments present supported the adoption of the World Anti-Doping Code. The Copenhagen Declaration signed by governments was a non–legally binding statement of political intention by each government to find the appropriate means of making the code the basis of its own fight against doping in sport. It was not an overwhelming commitment, but the governments assured us that it amounted to a political promise that would be taken seriously by any government that signed it.

Now, at last, we had a single code in place. It was little short of a miracle that the process had brought us this far this quickly. But WADA's adoption of the code was only the beginning. The code meant nothing until the sports

Why Do We Need to Regulate Doping?

movement and governments acted to incorporate it into their own rules. Something like this is not too difficult for the sports movement, since there are regular meetings of the IFs and NOCs, at which decisions of this nature can be made. Since we were already in 2003, it seemed appropriate that the sports movement undertake to have the code implemented as part of each stakeholder's rules by the beginning of 2004, but, in any event, not later than the opening ceremony of the Athens Olympics later that year. Once again, this schedule was too quick for the governments, who said that the intergovernmental mechanism (on which they had not yet decided) would be too complicated to be accomplished in such a short period. They asked for a delay, until the 2006 Olympic Winter Games in Turin. There was little alternative but to agree, although some sports leaders grumbled aloud about why they had to adopt the code so quickly if the governments did not. I must say that I had no sympathy whatsoever for this kind of whining. These leaders had their own responsibilities to make sure their sports were clean, whether or not governments were willing to assist them in their efforts. It was annoying to see them casting about for any excuse to not do their own jobs. No wonder we had so many doping problems.

On the sports side, the adoption generally went very well. The IOC again led the way, adopting the code at its 2003 session in Prague. It went even further, amending the Olympic Charter to provide that only sports governed by international federations that had adopted and implemented the code could be or remain on the program of the Olympic Games. In cases like hockey, for example, when the sport is played at the Olympics, it is under the IIHF rules, with national teams, and has no relation to the NHL. This was a very important development, one that Samaranch, despite being the acknowledged strongman of

CHAPTER SEVEN

international sport, had never been willing to do during his twenty-one years as IOC president. This change, now in place, provided real leverage in dealing with even the largest IFs. They remained entirely free to decide whether or not they would adopt and implement the code, so they could not complain about anyone impinging on their autonomy.

The only thing now was that there would be major consequences arising from a failure to adopt the code—they would no longer be part of the Olympic Games. Imagine an IF president announcing at a press conference that his or her sport would no longer be on the Olympic program because, in its wisdom and exercise of its precious autonomy, the IF refused to adopt anti-doping rules approved by the entire Olympic Movement and the governments of all five continents. Imagine how long that president and executive would remain in office once the membership learned of this—especially when they discovered that, as in most countries where governments provide sport funding, such funding is usually directed at Olympic sports and the inevitable outcome at the national level would be the disappearance of such funding, not to mention the international showcase of the Olympic Games. Imagine being the president's press attaché and having to draft an answer to the question as to how the IF could possibly have made such a stupid decision. A further consequence of not being part of the Olympic Games was that any such federations would cease to share in the television and other revenues derived from the Games. The same impact would also occur where a NOC chose not to adopt and implement the code. So, even if there may not have been total conviction involved regarding doping in their sports, there was at least self-interest. One by one, starting at the beginning of 2004, the IFs and NOCs took the necessary

Why Do We Need to Regulate Doping?

steps to adopt the code. Cycling was the very last, waiting until the day before the opening ceremony of the Olympics to act. There was speculation that they wanted to run a final Tour de France under the pre-code rules.

Moving from the sports movement to governments, they eventually decided to create an international convention under the aegis of UNESCO (since doping fell within its general scope of activity) and they set about negotiating its terms. We, as WADA, kept track of the negotiations and made sure we were present when there were negotiating sessions so that the negotiators, who often had no idea about doping in sport and the context of the convention they were negotiating, could have access to whatever sport-related and doping-related expertise they needed. The rest of the Olympic Movement was not much involved in the process, despite our several requests for assistance. After months and months of asking for comments (so that they could be incorporated into the negotiations leading to the final draft convention that would be studied by governments), they came forward with a list of complaints, long after the final version of the convention had been circulated to the member countries of UNESCO in March 2005 and virtually on the eve of the conference, far too late to have been of any use whatsoever.

It was vital for us that the convention have enough teeth to ensure that the Code remained the basis of the fight against doping in sport and that the means of resolving sports-related doping issues was delegated to CAS. One of our big problems was to be certain that, every time the List of prohibited substances and methods was amended, we did not have to come back to UNESCO and start the whole process of negotiation all over again. This would not have bothered the bureaucrats all that much—they love meetings in exotic places—but it would have been a

CHAPTER SEVEN

nightmare for us, since the List changes every year. The negotiators said it was impossible for governments to sign off, sight unseen, on changes that WADA might make from time to time. So, we settled on a mechanism that would preserve the fundamental sovereignty of states, which was that, as we adopted changes to the List, we would notify UNESCO, which in turn would notify the member states of the changes. If a member state did not accept the change, which it is perfectly free to decide, it would have a certain amount of time to signify its dissent. Failing notification of dissent, the member state would be considered to have accepted the amended List.

The careful shepherding of the process and the efforts we made to get as many political commitments as we could eventually paid off. On October 19, 2005, at the thirty-third UNESCO General Conference in Paris, the participating 191 member states, of which 120 actually sponsored the re-solution, unanimously adopted the International Convention against Doping in Sport. It was one of the highlights of the International Year for Physical Education and Sports. This action provides, of course, only the framework. In order for the convention to come into force, it must be ratified by thirty countries, accomplished by depositing instruments of ratification, acceptance, approval and accession. The first to file its notice of ratification was Sweden. The second was Canada.

One problem that we had not anticipated was the delay between the conference decision and the delivery by UNESCO of formal copies of the convention in the six official languages of UNESCO, each of which had to be individually approved by the UNESCO lawyers. Naturally, this takes longer than anyone can understand. This general delay did not leave enough time for the governmental processes of ratification to be completed by the end of

Why Do We Need to Regulate Doping?

December, so we were not able to say that the convention was legally in force at the time of the Games in February 2006. This had no practical impact on the Games, because the World Anti-Doping Code was to be applied there regardless of whether the convention was in place at that time. It did, however, give the sports movement an opportunity to criticize governments for failing to move quickly enough. It will probably take most of 2006 to get the necessary ratifications in place to give the convention its formal status as such.

GIVE US THE TOOLS

If you are going to take on a job that requires serious work, you have to be sure you have the right tools for the job. And, as Abraham Lincoln once observed, if he had seven hours to chop down a tree, he would use six of them to sharpen the axe.

As 2005 ended and 2006 began, the world became equipped with the structural tools it needs to deal with all facets of doping in sport. The same rules will be applied by sport organizations and governments and, for the first time in history, all of the stakeholders necessary for coordinating the fight against doping in sport are together, at the same table, at the same time and with the same objectives. These are, however, just the tools. How they will be used and how cooperatively they will be used remain huge questions. Monitoring compliance with the promises will be a major responsibility for WADA on the code side of the equation, and for governments on the convention side. But, one way or another, we are a long way ahead of where we were before WADA was created. If I had said, at the press conference in Lausanne in 1999, that within six years we would have

CHAPTER SEVEN

in place an active organization, staffed and jointly funded by the Olympic Movement and governments, that we would have a single set of anti-doping rules unanimously approved by all stakeholders, that 191 countries would have approved an international convention against doping in sport and that there would be agreement on a single forum for dispute resolution and that this was the CAS, I would probably have been taken away for some delusion-reducing medical treatment.

08 Playing Fair, and Willing to Prove It

When you sign your multimillion-dollar contract, when you show up at the competition, when you look your fellow competitor in the eye, when you sign an autograph for an admiring kid, you are affirming that you play by the rules and that you are prepared to demonstrate this at any time, night or day, in or out of competition. If you are not willing to live by these rules, nobody is forcing you to participate. If you don't like proving you play fair, then don't play.

I think the world needs lawyers to help protect people from possible abuse by the state and other citizens. I am a lawyer, and I love my profession for that reason. In criminal matters, I believe in the presumption of innocence, the right to remain silent and in requiring the state, before it can deprive someone of liberty, or worse, life, to prove guilt beyond all reasonable doubt, in front of a jury of the accused's peers. These are hallmarks of a civilized society,

CHAPTER EIGHT

and the legal profession has as vital a role in administering justice as do the authorities and the courts.

But not all legal matters in society at large involve criminal conduct. Cheating in sport is not a criminal offence, although some criminal codes do outlaw some of these behaviors. It is a breach of the deal made between the players as to the rules that they agree will apply to themselves and the games they play. Athletes also agree among themselves on what happens if someone breaks those rules. There can be penalties, loss of possession of a ball, loss of position on the field of play, being thrown out of a game or event and so on. The nature and extent of the penalties are determined by the participants. Some are minor, while others are major. They are, however, sport rules, not rules of society, so generally they are not criminal in nature. This is an important distinction and one that is often not understood by the media and other commentators on what happens when sanctions are imposed on those breaking the rules.

When athletes appear on the field of play for any game, they are making a positive statement that they have complied with all the rules, before and during the game or event. One of the sport rules is that athletes will not use or do anything on the list of prohibited substances or doping methods. So, as an athlete, when you sign a multimillion-dollar contract, it is an affirmation that you will play by the rules. When you show up at the stadium, you are declaring to your fellow competitors and to the public at large that you will be following the rules that apply to everyone. When you sign an autograph for a young, star-smitten fan, you are assuring him or her that you are a real hero—not a miserable cheat. Remember the famous "Say it ain't so, Joe" of the 1919 Chicago Black Sox? How many of today's stars, especially in professional sports, could look a kid in the eye and say, honestly, "It ain't so, kid—I did this without cheating."

Another aspect is that the players agree to demonstrate that they are adhering to the rules by submitting to tests, both in and out of competition. The players and the public alike are aware of this agreement. Testing out of competition can, and should, be done at any time and any place. Everyone knows that "smart" cheaters can always arrange to be "clean" on game day. It's the off-season, the preparation phase, that is particularly important for this purpose. The sports community also agrees that the standard applied for doping purposes is one of what is called "strict liability." This means that the doping offense is complete and final if the presence of the prohibited substance is found in the athlete's system, or if there is evidence of the use or attempted use of a prohibited method (such as blood doping). It is not necessary to prove that there was any intention to improve performance; nor does it matter whether or not it was effective. It's doping. Period.

Now, here is where the lawyers have interfered with the sport rules and where sports organizations have been taken along for the ride. The lawyers insist that their athlete clients are entitled to complete confidentiality, despite their own agreement that they are willing to be tested on a 24/7/365 basis. Some lawyers argue that no one should be entitled to know whether an athlete has been tested or not and no one should be entitled to know whether an athlete has tested positive. These lawyers act as if some sacred constitutional right has been born and needs to be protected, when all that is at stake is whether an athlete is, or is not, following one of the freely agreed-upon rules of sport. It would be like arguing that you should be be able to keep secret your boxing weight, or that your bat is corked, or that your hockey stick is curved too much, or that your bobsled has heated runners, or that your shot put is hollowed out, or that your racing bicycle is lighter than the specified limit—

CHAPTER EIGHT

that all are strictly private matters about which no one else should be informed. But when you agree to compete in sport, you agree to abide by the established rules, and you agree to give up all privacy rights in this regard. Your competitors and the public have a right to know whether you do or you do not comply with the rules.

In late December 2005, American skier Bode Miller was fined because he refused to allow his ski boots to be measured to see if they complied with the FIS rules. He said it was a ridiculous rule. Besides, he said that he had already taken off his boots, so it would be impossible to tell whether he could have adjusted them any way he wanted. The rule, however, provided that they be measured while he was still wearing them, because no manipulation could occur until after they had been removed. His personal wall of noise could not draw attention away from the fact that he refused to allow his boots to be measured, a rule he accepted in order to be able to stand at the top of the hill in the first place. This is the same Miller who insists that athletes should be allowed to use performance-enhancing drugs and who pouts publicly that no one wants to debate the issue with him, despite the absolute rejection of his position by many of his fellow athletes. I believe he has a constitutional right to make a complete fool of himself, if he so chooses. If all these troubling rules offend him so much that he feels unjustifiably put-upon, he should, as a Texan friend of mine used to say, not let the door hit his ass on the way out.

I notice, with resignation but no surprise, that there are some American lawyers ready to argue that compulsory drug testing in sport is a breach of the protection, provided by the Fourth Amendment of the U.S. Constitution, against unreasonable search and seizure. I suppose this sort of challenge is inevitable, especially in a country that boasts the largest collection of lawyers on the face of the planet.

Playing Fair, and Willing to Prove It

The sport that probably uses this argument the most is—surprise, surprise—Major League Baseball (MLB), led by its players' union, the MLBPA. It wants minimal testing, if any, and minimal sanctions, although it has finally backed, under congressional pressure, into sanctions that are somewhat better, with a fifty-game suspension for the first offence, 100 games for the second and lifetime for the third. MLB either just doesn't get it, or is institutionally blind to what is going on within the sport and all around them. They have an agreement among themselves and their players that the players will not use drugs, and the existence of such an agreement is regularly trumpeted in public. There are, however, many players in MLB who are clearly using or have used performance-enhancing drugs. Among them are, to name but a few, Mark McGwire, Rafael Palmeiro and Barry Bonds and, more recently, Jason Grimsley and others whom he may implicate.

There is an agreed-upon right to test, even though it almost seems designed to be sure that no one with an IQ in excess of room temperature is ever caught. And when someone does stumble into the deliberately primitive trap, MLB has a system of sanctions that makes it clear that there is no urgency whatsoever to stamp out the practice of doping. We're talking here about players in the national sport of the United States, who are role models for the public—including its impressionable youth—and who make extremely good livings in the process, playing a genuine game in accordance with the rules of baseball. In fact, knowing there is widespread drug use without serious penalties is a deception on the public by owners and players alike. I would love to watch the legal cross-hairs of a good judge center on the open mouth of a lawyer complaining in court that his drug-using client has had his constitutional rights violated because he was subjected to the test that exposed him as a cheater.

CHAPTER EIGHT

But what about the rights of an athlete whose opponent has promised to play by the rules of the game, who has been cheated out of winning by someone who is secretly using performance-enhancing drugs? How would you like your child, your neighbor's child or anyone, for that matter, to lose a race by a few inches, a tenth of a second, because someone cheated? How would you like to see years of effort, devoted to becoming the best they can be in their sport, trivialized because someone who has no respect for the game, for his opponents and, ultimately, for himself, deliberately used drugs that would give him that extra advantage? These people, and those around them who help them to cheat, are the sociopaths of sport. They need to be exposed and removed from the competitions they are tainting, so that sport can be conducted by the rules everyone agreed upon in the first place. The alternative is that sport slips into the downward cycle where everyone is forced to out-cheat the cheaters. Responsible parents, coaches and athletes will end up turning their backs on unfair play and the risks of permanent damage to health. Whatever the activity may become, it will not be sport.

Let's take a step back and review the MLB situation. We are not dealing with criminal or penal law; we are dealing with an agreement between players, who promise each other, as well as their fans (who ultimately pay their salaries), that they will not use drugs in their sport and who agree, as part of that participation, that they can be tested to make sure that they are adhering to their promises and following the rules. Don't forget that this is all voluntary. If an individual does not agree with the sport rules, he does not need to participate. The freedom to opt out is available at all times. It is not like society in general, where one must comply with the laws of the land.

So, this is not a plea to kill all the lawyers, but simply to keep them in their place and not allow them to defend drug use in sport as if they were protecting constitutional rights in criminal prosecutions. As to the apparently inevitable constitutional challenge, whether in baseball or some other sport, I should, perhaps, rephrase this and say, let's get it over with. Let the argument be made and be considered by the courts. Once a final decision is rendered, the argument can be thrown on the dump heap of sport history as yet another unpersuasive effort to weaken the fight against doping in sport.

CRIME AND PUNISHMENT

Doping is cheating, and there must be consequences for that. Serious penalties for doping will show that cheaters are not welcome and will act as a deterrent to discourage others from cheating.

Until the adoption of the World Anti-Doping Code in 2003, the penalties for doping in sport, and even agreement on the substances that ought to be prohibited, were all over the map. In some sports, the penalty for the first infraction was a lifetime suspension, which was obviously too severe a penalty, and the federations knew such bans would likely not stand up in the normal courts should athletes challenge them. The penalty allowed them to sound tough, knowing that there was a way out for the athletes. Other sports imposed a four-year sanction, with which some courts also disagreed. This led the federations concerned to routinely reduce penalties to eighteen months upon application by the athlete. Still others had variable sanctions, usually much lighter, often to the point that they were a joke. In many cases, the penalties were given no publicity, so any deterrent

CHAPTER EIGHT

effect was completely lost. This patchwork of approaches to doping sent a mixed message and did nothing to focus attention on it, or to underline the importance of getting a handle on it.

The penalty imposed for breaking a rule must reflect the seriousness of the offense. Criminal courts today would not sentence a person to life imprisonment for stealing a loaf of bread, any more than they would impose a two-week sentence for a violent armed robbery. In the process of developing the Code, we consulted many international legal experts about the proposed standard two-year penalty for a first serious doping offense. The consensus was that barring an athlete from competition for a minimum of two years was reasonable and did not violate any human rights legislation, especially where there was some built-in flexibility to consider truly exceptional circumstances and adjust the sanctions if appropriate.

Thus far, despite some negative comments, mostly from international federations, the general agreement is that a two-year sanction for a serious doping offence is fair. The Court of Arbitration for Sport (CAS) has agreed, even pointing out that such a sentence is more likely to be effective in dealing with doping than lighter sanctions would be. As I am writing this, international federations are meeting together to try to find some way to reduce the penalties in future. This is completely off message. I bet they will encounter stiff—and well deserved—resistance from others in the fight against doping in sport, including athletes, the IOC, national Olympic committees and governments.

Minimum sentences can be reduced in certain cases, and a positive test may be ruled as "no fault" on the part of the athlete. This means that if you were attacked by a squad of terrorists and injected with an anabolic steroid on the way to your event, and subsequently tested positive, your result in the competition would be cancelled but because it was not your fault you would not face further penalties. The definition of no "significant" fault, which could reduce the penalty by half, or one year, is being ironed out over time as the CAS deals with specific cases. In the case of Zack Lund, for example, he was considered not to be at significant fault because he had declared that he was taking the masking agent on his doping control forms and no one in authority had apparently told him that the hair restorer contained a masking agent.

But an athlete cannot expect a reduced penalty because of mere carelessness. Nor should the size of an athlete's salary and the amount of money he or she might lose if sanctioned be a consideration. Frankly, I think that if you are making a lot of money on the pretext that you are competing fairly and within the rules and then you are exposed as a cheater, you deserve to lose all the money you would have made during your period of suspension. Maybe you should even return the money you earned while you were cheating. This is what happened to Dwain Chambers.

In 2006, the International Association of Athletics Federation (IAAF), which governs track and field, ruled that former European sprint champion Dwain Chambers must repay the US$230,615 prize money he won while using steroids. Chambers tested positive twice for THG and was banned in 2004 for two years. The IAAF ruled that he would not be allowed to compete again until he repays the money. This action by the IAAF was unique. We can only hope that it is precedent-setting for other sports associations and governing bodies. This would surely make athletes think twice about cheating. But no matter how thin you slice it, the basic principle remains—it is every athlete's responsibility to ensure that prohibited substances are not used.

CHAPTER EIGHT

RESPONSIBILITY OF THE ATHLETE'S SUPPORT STAFF

Coaches, doctors and officials have a great responsibility to their athletes. If they are involved in doping, they should face even greater penalties than the athletes. They should lose the right to coach or practice. End of discussion

An athlete's support staff—coaches, doctors, officials and so on—can create even more problems. My view is that these people have an even greater responsibility than the athletes, and, if they are involved in doping, they should face even tougher penalties. It's always frustrating to see coaches from the former East Germany reappear in other countries, which coincidentally achieve much better results than normally expected. These coaches, who had previously perverted sport, not only were not punished, but they were allowed to continue with their old tricks in a new setting. They should have lost the right to coach, period. At the very least, they should have been prevented from continuing to use illicit methods. Sadly, their new employers seem to want success above all and are not willing to look too closely at how the results are obtained. There was a lot of publicity when Tim Montgomery and Marion Jones were considering the possibility of putting themselves under the care of the notorious East German coach Ekkart Arbeit. When the outrage became generalized, they changed to the idea of using Ben Johnson's coach, Charlie Francis. Eventually they also abandoned that idea, but the message was that they, and other athletes, are willing to go where they know that success will follow, even if there is a history of drug-assisted success.

Coaches who cheat should be exposed and banned from coaching. The same should be true with doctors who administer performance-enhancing drugs. Romanian gymnast Andrea Raducan lost her gold medal in gymnastics at Sydney after she tested positive for pseudoephedrine. Her team doctor had given her cold tablets containing the stimulant. Fortunately, he will not be accredited at future Olympic Games, but he probably doesn't care. He and other doctors willing to do the same thing continue to practice medicine as licensed physicians and no professional disciplinary action whatsoever is imposed.

We have been unsuccessful in getting consensus among medical doctors to condemn, clearly, publicly and unequivocally, the use of performance-enhancing drugs in sport. In my view, the medical profession hides behind the idea of patient autonomy, which is a fancy way of saying that what the patient wants, he gets, even if the doctor knows that the patient wants it for the express purpose of cheating in sport. Some doctors justify themselves by saying that athletes would probably use the prohibited substances anyway, so it is better that they do so under medical supervision. How hypocritical!

Perhaps the most famous doping case of all was Ben Johnson, who tested positive for steroids following his extraordinary Olympic victory in the 100 meters at Seoul. He was disqualified and his medal taken away. A few months later, I participated at a conference where a panel of medical "ethicists" discussed a variety of ethical issues that cropped up in sport. At the end of the discussion, I suggested from the floor a hypothetical scenario as follows. A patient comes to them and says, "Hi, my name is Ben Johnson. I am a pretty good runner and I am training for the Olympics. But I don't think that I can win unless I use anabolic steroids. I have to tell you that they are completely illegal in the Olympics. I don't have a medical condition, so, for me, they have no therapeutic value at all. They will simply help me to train harder and run faster,

CHAPTER EIGHT

so I want you to prescribe them for me, even though they are prohibited." I asked them, as medical practitioners and ethicists, what they would do in the circumstances. To my absolute astonishment, each of them said they would prescribe the drugs. On what possible basis, I asked. "Autonomy of the patient," they intoned.

Patient autonomy, surely, cannot be the complete answer. At the very least, doctors have some kind of duty to live by the Hippocratic oath, to do no harm. Choosing a "treatment" or allowing a patient to choose something that does obvious harm is, in my view, a breach of that oath. I do not believe that a medical doctor can be unaware that a patient under his or her charge is using prohibited substances for non-therapeutic purposes. I suppose it is possible that occasionally a doctor may be fooled, especially if the athlete shops around and obtains prescriptions from several doctors, but this would be the exception and not the rule. There are too many cases in which cheating in sport has been made possible with the active help, and even encouragement, of medical practitioners.

I realized then that the medical profession had abandoned any pretence of being an ethical leader in sport. Frankly, it seemed, from a professional perspective, that doctors would be as likely to assist cheaters as they would be to help keep competition pure. I found this attitude as disappointing as it was inexplicable. I did not, however, want to suggest that the medical profession was devoid of ethics. I was sure that many organizations and professional associations had developed ethical rules regarding appropriate actions in this field. My question was whether these professional organizations enforced the rules that they themselves had adopted. I suggested to the medical panel that they did not. If they did not regulate themselves in such matters, then it might become necessary to look elsewhere and to have third-party enforcement. Does this sound familiar?

The same difficulty had been encountered with the pharmaceutical industry. It cannot help but be aware that products are being acquired and used for purposes that are not therapeutic. But the industry does nothing to regulate the sale or monitor the distribution of the products for such uses. Profit seems to be a greater good than ethics. I called—with a spectacular lack of success—on the pharmaceutical industry to help us promote the ethical values of sport. I hoped as well that there would be those within the scientific research community who could speak out against the use of athletes as subjects for purposes of developing performance-enhancing substances and methods that are so clearly antithetical to the spirit of sport. There was a particularly disappointing uptake on the ethical aspects of cheating. It was going to be a long and difficult road ahead.

Fortunately, with the new international convention against doping in sport, we finally have the possibility of getting at such unethical professionals. Within sport, there was nothing we could do to discipline them from a professional perspective. But now, governments are taking a stand as part of their commitment to the fight against doping in sport. They have the capacity to make it mandatory that the professional organizations include in their professional codes of conduct that doctors will not administer performance-enhancing drugs or methods unless the proposed use is genuinely therapeutic in nature. Doctors should have a "know your patient" obligation—along the lines that now apply in the banking and investment fields—that will prevent them from prescribing such prohibited substances or using prohibited methods with athletes. The penalties should be severe enough to act as a deterrent, and infractions, plus the disciplinary sanctions, should be made public. They should be shamed into stopping! This is just one of many ways in which governments can give content to their part in this fight. Add to that the kind of investigations that uncovered the Balco and Spanish conspiracies, and the potential to discover and stop doping activities, especially possession and trafficking, in addition to use, becomes much more exciting.

BEYOND PUNISHMENT: CHANGING ATTITUDES

In the long run, it is a matter of changing attitudes through education and creating a climate that understands that it is important for sport to be drug-free.

For the moment, we have to continue to rely on a combination of tests and sanctions. With luck, the penalties will have an impact, especially if they are severe enough to act as a deterrent.

But punishment is not the only answer to the problem of doping in sport. It is not even the most important response, although it must be a part of the overall solution. In the long run, it is a matter of changing attitudes through education and creating a climate that understands that it is important for sport to be drug-free. I think back to the days when I first got my driver's license. I did not bother to use seat belts, even after they became mandatory. I was young and immortal, and the possibility of my being injured or killed in an accident never figured in my mind for an instant. Accidents happened to other people, not to me. And it was not the occasional fine or points deducted from my license that eventually changed my attitude. It was the gradual realization that it was unutterably stupid to be driving without a seat belt. Now, I am at the stage of being intensely uncomfortable if I am in a car without fastening my seat belt. That is the type of attitude shift I hope we can create in sport.

This is exactly what happens to athletes who use the performance-enhancing drugs and methods. They are convinced they will never be caught and, where Balco-like situations exist, are reinforced in that view by the Contes and Korchemnys of the world who are complicit with them. Don't worry, they are assured, the testers will never find it. If warned of the health risks, they are similarly convinced that they will not be among those who will be affected. Too many athletes are like those who answered a questionnaire that asked a question along the lines of "If you were to take a certain drug that would guarantee that you would win the next Olympics, but would almost certainly die within five years as a result, would you take the drug?" An extraordinary number of them answered that they would take the drug. The bad stuff would not happen to them, only the good would, like the Olympic gold medal. It would be some other fool, some loser, who would be dead.

Athletes are, for the most part, positive thinkers. That is an important part of their success and it reinforces their efforts to improve their performance. They feed off the positive attitude and do as much as possible to eliminate any negative thoughts. They can easily fool or persuade themselves that taking drugs is not "wrong." How could it be cheating, they say, if everyone is doing it? So what is known to be wrong gets pulled and twisted into the reverse of what it really is. Many athletes who get caught for doping have genuinely convinced themselves that they were doing nothing wrong and have been able to work up righteous indignation when confronted with the evidence of the doping. This ability to fool themselves is not surprising—people do this all the time in many aspects of ordinary life. It underlines the importance of proper

CHAPTER EIGHT

coaching and parental oversight in young athletes, to provide an understanding of the ethical foundations of sport, a gut comprehension that it is only worth doing if it is done for the right reason. The concept of self-respect is absolutely vital: I will not cheat—it is unworthy of me and I respect myself too much to stoop to such behaviour. This requires us to find ways to break through the unjustified optimism or the rationalization, to get the athletes to focus on the genuine risks, both medical and ethical, arising from doping. How do we make it real for them? Some of this we do with our Athlete Outreach programs at Olympic Games and other major events, where we have direct contact with them and a chance to explain what doping does to them and to sport. It is always interesting to see how little many of them actually know much about the subject, which is both encouraging and disturbing. Encouraging because it tends to mean that they are not, themselves, involved in doping; disturbing because it means that they can be more easily manipulated by those on whom they depend for support. At least with our outreach, we can alert them to the kinds of doping that may be out there, to watch for symptoms and for the types of blandishment they might encounter. Some sensitization is achieved through educational programs, both in print and on our web site, some at international meetings of sport leaders, some through public speaking and media appearances. The key is a combination of repetition, consistency and reaching audiences around the world, not exclusively the athletes. You need leverage and have to find it where you can in order to have your message delivered on occasion by someone else who can, in turn, influence the athlete.

Realistically, however, even if the educational programs are successful beyond our wildest dreams, we will have to continue to have both elements—testing and sanctions as well as education—as part of the arsenal.

09 Pro Sports I: Baseball, Football and Basketball

Professional sport is a business. The objective is to make money. Those involved will do whatever they have to do to make money, including rule changes, artificial stoppages of play, encouraging violence on the field of play and creating "stars." They wouldn't dare say that they encourage or tolerate drug use, so they have rules against it. But it is mostly window dressing.

You would think that sports authorities, as well as public authorities, would be concerned about the rash of deaths and debilitating injuries among young high-performance athletes. Why are deaths occurring with such frequency? Why are they occurring in sports that are known to have drug problems? Is there not some connection between drug use in the sport and the untimely deaths? What could be done to study the problem and to reduce or eliminate the use of drugs?

CHAPTER NINE

These are all questions that seem self-evident to anyone who thinks about the problem for more than five minutes. But, for far too long, no one in authority did anything. They looked the other way or simply denied that there was a drug problem, even when there was mounting evidence to the contrary. The public was also willing to swallow the bland assurances that were issued by the leagues. Politicians paid only sporadic attention to the issue. In most countries, the professional leagues are acknowledged to be private enterprises, subject to the general laws of the land but otherwise left on their own, free to regulate their activities as they see fit, without active government interference. But, when you look a bit closer, you see that they like to suck and whistle at the same time. In fact, professional leagues have begged for government exemptions from some laws, such as the anti-trust legislation in the United States. The United States is not the only country with this general attitude, although its leagues, teams, players and owners are perhaps the most well known.

Professional sports are businesses. They exist to make money for the owners and the players, and they depend on the willingness of fans to buy tickets. Those fans not in the stadiums watch the game on television, which encourages broadcasters and their sponsors to pay significant amounts to attract fan attention. If the fans want more violence, that is what they get. If the broadcasters need more time to advertise their television sponsors, the rules of the games are changed to allow for more commercial breaks. It is simply a matter of trying to get the balance right and trying not to do anything that will cause commercial interest to diminish. Schedules get longer, rules change to permit more exciting, higher-scoring games and equipment is improved to allow for higher impact—whatever it takes to make more money. Stars are created and promoted to allow uninformed fans unable

Pro Sports I: Baseball, Football and Basketball

to follow the game as a whole to identify with an individual. State and municipal authorities fall all over themselves to attract professional teams, and taxpayer dollars subsidize the stadiums where owners and players make their money. Corporate resources are tapped for luxury accommodation and entertainment packages at playing field venues. It is a wonderful money-making machine. And it has one splendid advantage for the owners. All they have to do is pay a current market value for their inventory—the players—without any responsibility (or cost) for the development of the talent that makes their businesses profitable. And, for public relations purposes, they occasionally pay some lip service to doping-free sport.

There is a general similarity among all the leagues, both economically and in their approach to drug use. Some are more successful financially than others, and some have a slightly more enlightened approach to drug use. From time to time, the professional leagues seem to be willing to take some flack from governments and the media about drug use in their backyards. After all, they know that, in the long run, nothing is likely to happen to them, so the seven-day tempest in the teapot is a price they are willing pay. Outside the government sphere, they can be more controlling. One of the ways they minimize bad press is by denying access to overly critical media, a strategy that has been fairly effective. No one speaks about it—that would be bad press. The United States Olympic Committee (USOC) regularly refused Olympic credentials to journalists who were critical of it. The Union Cycliste Internationale (UCI) president, Hein Verbruggen, told me he used to refuse to speak with a reporter from *L'Equipe* who was critical of the UCI and of the sport. He regularly refers to me as a "sheriff from the wild west" because I have dared to bring attention to the drug problems in cycling, forgetting, of course, that the sheriff is the good guy who catches the bad guys. And a sheriff with a quick draw is more likely to prosper than one who is slow off the mark—when you deal with cheaters, don't forget they have already made the first move! Reporters have been banned from locker rooms or clubhouses for being critical. I do not make a habit of remembering their names, but recall it happening on many occasions. Anyone who speaks out from within a league, someone like José Canseco in MLB, is dismissed as a crank and ostracized. The leagues seem willing to endure the occasional heat and then go back to business as usual—seeing, hearing and speaking no drug evil. That is why the problem has become worse and more widespread.

MAJOR LEAGUE BASEBALL

> *MLB's "get tough" policy on drug use was a complete joke. If a player tested positive for steroids five times, he might face up to a year's suspension. It's sort of like holding up the same liquor store five times in a row and getting off with a maximum of a year of community service!*

Take Major League Baseball (MLB), for example. In early 2003 an apparently perfectly healthy young player, Steve Bechler, collapsed and died during the Baltimore Orioles' spring training. Following his death, investigators found indications of drug use—ephedrine. MLB, naturally, denied that there was a drug problem in baseball.

Public pressure led the U.S. Congress to inquire into the matter and to invite MLB to give evidence. MLB resolutely, and predictably, denied that baseball had a drug problem. Congress did not buy it, and MLB reluctantly agreed that it would conduct tests. At the end of the season, if the league found that five percent or more of the players had tested positive, it would acknowledge that there was a problem and take steps to deal with it. To make sure it was "independent," MLB managed the whole process itself. Outside observers were not invited. After all, MLB had said there was no problem.

It sounds responsive, doesn't it? But look at what actually happened. First, the only tests MLB did were for anabolic steroids. They left out other drugs—such as stimulants, human growth hormone and EPO—which were known to be in active use among the players. Next, the players were all warned, repeatedly, that they would be tested, but they were assured that they would be tested only during the season. Everyone knows that steroids are often used in the off-season, with the benefits continuing into the season.

And now for the tests. This supposedly rigorous examination into possible drug use in MLB was set up so that, if a player tested positive—even after all the warnings of impending tests—he was able to have a second chance later. It gets worse. If the player managed to clear his system by the time of the second test and produced a negative result, the earlier positive test was not even counted in the total when calculating the five percent! Even with this outrageous process, at the end of the season, MLB was forced to admit that the positive tests had totalled well over five percent, the self-serving threshold that the league itself had set as an arbitrary standard. Naturally, no names of players who tested positive were released. Maybe they thought that it would be too embarrassing for the players, since failing a drug test after all the warnings and a chance for a second test would have been akin to failing an intelligence test as well.

As a result, MLB was left with no alternative but to change its anti-drug policies for the following season. Their own results made it clear that there was indeed a drug use problem in baseball. (Of course, everyone except MLB already knew this.) Adding further insult to the intelligence

CHAPTER NINE

of the public, MLB announced a firm step forward. For the first offense—and remember that part of the official deal in baseball is that there is no use of drugs—there would be a warning and counselling. A warning? What did anyone need to be warned about? Counselling? About not getting caught? A second offense (still only for steroids) would result in a fine of up to $10,000, which was nothing more than walking-around money for a player in MLB. It would not be until a *fifth* positive test that the drug-using player might face up to a year's suspension. It's sort of like holding up the same liquor store five times in a row and getting off with a maximum of a year of community service! An Olympic athlete would have been suspended for up to two years for a first offense and for life for a second offense.

MLB then had the gall to proclaim this a victory—the end of the drug problem in baseball. It publicly congratulated itself on having managed a breakthrough in the fight against drugs in baseball. A new collective bargaining agreement between the MLB and its Players Association was quickly signed so that the deal would be put to bed and not be re-opened until the end of the convenient new contract period. The players and management marched off into the sunset, all but holding hands. However, the agreement was for steroids only, and the league was not yet "ready" to consider stimulants and other drugs that were known to be in wide use. They would not have to reopen talks on these drugs until the next round of collective bargaining, now years in the future. The "get tough" policy was a complete joke and an insult to the intelligence of anyone with an IQ higher than room temperature. But they did not get away with it. There was enough public outrage and ridicule to attract further congressional attention. You know that you have been characterized as ridiculous when talk show hosts and cartoonists begin to use you as the butt of their jokes.

Pro Sports I: Baseball, Football and Basketball

I was listening to the 2004 State of the Union address of President George W. Bush, the annual flow of carefully negotiated and nuanced verbiage, beginning to wonder whether this was the All-Time Dullest or at least within the Top-Ten Dullest addresses, when, all of a sudden, from out of nowhere, the issue of drug use in professional sports in the United States was raised to the top of the policy issues facing the nation. The president of the United States was calling on professional sports to clean up their drug problems, with the implicit threat that if they did not do so voluntarily, it would be done for them. Who knows what combination of factors led to this? Perhaps the presidential advisors felt it necessary to respond to the growing perception of the United States as a country not serious about doping in sport, in the professional leagues and in amateur sport as well, especially with the Balco revelations. Perhaps it was nothing more than an election gambit. The most important fact, however, was that it was now in front of the American public as a national issue.

There are many reasons why this was an important milestone. The fact that it was part of the State of the Union address was especially significant, since the issue had never made it that far up the presidential policy tree before. It was also official recognition that the problem existed and that those responsible for the professional sports had not been effective in dealing with it. Not only that, but the professional sports were now under a bright spotlight, one previously occupied only by the Olympic and amateur sports organizations, such as the USOC, National Collegiate Athletic Association (NCAA) and national governing bodies. For those of us active in the international field, it was important because the United States is a leader and can influence the behavior of others. When other professional leagues are pressed to address the problem of drug use, they

CHAPTER NINE

often ask why they should do something about doping when the American leagues do not. This is not a good excuse and rather childish, but I suppose they are quite used to passing the buck.

Bush acknowledging the drug problem was an important milestone for another reason. He did so in an election year. While some might (and did) say that it was nothing more than a grandstand play as part of his election campaign, what I thought it meant was that people would pay close attention to his follow-up actions. Doping certainly did not become a central theme in an otherwise uninspired and vindictive presidential campaign, but it remains an ongoing problem, and the congressional attention and hearings could be assisted by further expressions of presidential interest. His message was that professional sports should clean up their acts voluntarily, but if they did not, there might be other measures to be taken. Was he hinting that he would consider anti-doping legislation? I am not sure Bush would support specific legislation, given his general reluctance to interfere in anything that smacks of business, but who knows?

In the aftermath of the State of the Union address, the minimal efforts of MLB to address its problem attracted more congressional attention. In March 2005, it was invited to a hearing before a House committee. MLB was no more persuasive than before regarding its commitment to dealing with the doping problem in a meaningful manner. By now, the committee was clearly fed up with MLB's attitude and began to seriously consider the introduction of an anti-doping law.

As president of WADA, I used this as leverage to make sure that MLB was not the only professional sport to be targeted. Whenever possible, when interviewed, I made it clear that I thought the existing chummy MLB policy was a joke and that the public should not be fooled that

Pro Sports I: Baseball, Football and Basketball

the problem had been dealt with—and that the other professional sports were not much better, if at all.

More importantly, it was imperative to show that anabolic steroids (the only drugs on MLB's prohibited list) were not the only drugs used among the 1,500 or so MLB players. As I have said time and time again, steroids are only one class of drugs and there are many more used in MLB and other sports. Particularly cynical and dangerous, however, is the suggestion that only a few highly paid professional athletes are involved and at risk. Their leaders are fond of saying they are fully capable of assessing those risks and that the context is nothing more than an employer-employee relationship, which is their private business, and that it affects only them. Everyone should butt out and let them get on with their business in peace. What a load of baloney!

The fact of the matter is that the message we take away from the MLB position is that drugs work, they are tolerated at the highest level and if you want to get to the top you will have to use them. Players in Triple A leagues figure that if they want to get to the "show," they must use drugs. The clear signal is that the powers-that-be do not look carefully at their own rule books and, if they stumble (despite their best efforts not to) across drug use, they give nothing more than a wink and a nod, and a gentle slap on the wrist. So, to get to the top, the athletes down below use the drugs. The same process is repeated in Double A, in lesser leagues, college ball and even by younger and more impressionable players in high school ball. So, instead of there being a doping problem only at the MLB level, MLB's failure to deal with this issue helps to create a pyramid that may measure hundreds of thousands of young people at its base. Repeat the same example with the other professional sports and you have a problem that could affect millions of young people. This is a public policy issue that governments simply cannot ignore.

CHAPTER NINE

Senator John McCain has owned the drugs-in-sport issue in the Senate, and will no doubt manage the agenda if legislation reaches the Senate. McCain understands perfectly that we are well past the time when the leagues can be trusted to handle the drug problems internally. When I met with him in April 2005, he asked whether I thought that a good drug policy required an independent agency, such as WADA, to handle it. I said that I agreed with the idea of an independent agency, but thought the American public would be more comfortable with a U.S. organization, like the United States Anti-Doping Agency (USADA), as the independent agency responsible for American sports. This is not a time when the U.S. public has much enthusiasm for foreign agencies—of any kind—making judgments affecting Americans. McCain also understands the larger issue of the need within international sport to create a level playing field and to have a set of rules that will apply to everyone, no matter what country they come from and no matter what sport they practice. A unilateral U.S. policy on doping generally will not be sufficient, especially if it does not go as far as the rest of the world has already come. I suppose some point could be made that for U.S.-only sports, the U.S. could have its own rules, but the players do not only come from the U.S. and the influence of the U.S. leagues is such that if they take no action, others will be able to rationalize doing nothing as well. WADA offered to help the congressional leaders where we could, including testifying and giving suggestions as to lines of questioning that might assist the lawmakers to discover the extent of the professional inaction.

I believe there is little doubt that the approach to drug use in baseball as demonstrated by MLB was one of the factors that led to the IOC's decision in July 2005 to remove baseball from the Olympic program in 2012. It was not the

Pro Sports I: Baseball, Football and Basketball

only reason, since there is virtually no interest in baseball in Europe, where there is a concentration of IOC members. As well, the international baseball federation has done little to try to improve the quality of players in the Olympic tournaments, so the Olympic baseball tournament was well short of the best baseball in the world. But MLB's thumbing of its nose at the drug problem had a negative effect on the many IOC members and their willingness to allow it at future Olympic Games.

The attitude persists, even when MLB and the international baseball federation cooperated to organize the much-promoted 2006 World Baseball Classic, in which MLB players, players from other professional leagues and non-league players participated. This event was supposed to be organized under the rules contained in the World Anti-Doping Code, which meant that WADA would be able to perform out-of-competition testing on the players. When we tried to get a copy of the rules that would apply, the federation went dark. It refused our repeated requests to disclose the rules it would apply. It refused to provide WADA with the 2006 agreement that allowed us to test the players. It provided no results of the testing program during the Classic. Well after the event was over, we finally got the testing agreement. It had been signed in January and kept in a drawer until the event had finished and it was too late to have done anything. It is hard to imagine that this blatant stonewalling was unconnected with the participation of MLB and other professional league players.

One of the unfortunate side effects of the IOC decision regarding baseball was that the same shotgun blast resulted in the elimination of softball, reserved for women only, in which we had the best players at the Olympic Games and which does have a strong anti-doping policy. There is no evidence that MLB gives a damn about the fact that the

CHAPTER NINE

Olympics are now a closed book for young baseball players all over the world, not to mention the young women who play softball. Not only are the Olympics affected, but also the development of both sports in countries where government funding is focused on Olympic sports. These may have been unintended consequences arising from the MLB position on drugs, but they are nevertheless real.

It has always puzzled me somewhat that MLB has been willing to take a hard line against gambling on the part of its players but not with drug use, another form of cheating. Both gambling and drug use have an adverse impact on the integrity of the game, but only gambling seems to attract MLB's full attention. Both activities make the competition potentially artificial. In gambling, the effort by players or teams may not be real, and in doping, the players are not real, artificially juiced up so they can hit balls that are still rising as they leave the stadium. Pete Rose has been kept out of the Baseball Hall of Fame for gambling. I wonder what will happen to Mark McGwire, Sammy Sosa, Rafael Palmeiro and Barry Bonds, among others. McGwire imploded in front of the entire country with his refusal to talk about the "past," Palmeiro has become a laughing stock and Bonds has finally been exposed as a massive drug user, something the owners and players in MLB must have known all along. Double standards don't seem to bother the MLB. The litmus test may come as early as 2007 when Hall of Fame candidates are considered for admission. Then we will see how complicit the voters are in allowing baseball to be tainted by drugs. If MLB will not act, then maybe the public can express its condemnation of drug use in the sport. Maybe there can be two votes, one for the Hall of Fame and another for a Hall of Shame.

MLB's extraordinarily moronic treatment of the doping problem was so outrageous that it had triggered a further

Pro Sports I: Baseball, Football and Basketball

round of congressional attention during 2005. MLB was thoroughly beaten up, and it was clear that the U.S. Congress was ready to consider legislation, with support from both the Republicans and the Democrats. This finally got MLB to blink. Shortly after the end of the 2005 World Series, and just as mandatory-drug-testing legislation was about to be introduced and followed through on, MLB announced that yet another deal had been reached with the players. This was the first time that MLB tried to address some of the real issues that it had ignored in its previous "get tough" policies. The penalties were increased significantly, although they fall way short of what Olympic athletes face:

- A first positive test will result in a fifty-game suspension (less than a third of the regular season).
- A second positive test will result in a 100-game suspension.
- A third positive test will lead to a lifetime suspension, except that, when you read the fine print, it is not really a lifetime suspension, since the player can apply for reinstatement after two years and a decision to refuse reinstatement is subject to arbitration.

To be fair, this is progress of a sort, even if it cynically goes only as far as MLB thinks is necessary to keep Congress from passing an anti-doping law. From the silence in Congress, MLB judged it correctly—for the moment. The whole question of amphetamines and stimulants, which were not dealt with before by MLB, has now been addressed for the first time, albeit mildly in comparison with steroids, and only for 2006 and beyond. Testing would be mandatory, once during spring training (virtually useless, since the players know it is coming and know when spring training starts) and once more during the season, on a random

CHAPTER NINE

basis (whatever that means). However, there remains the possibility of further tests, even after the first random test. If the policy is to have any real credibility, there must also be complete integrity in the testing by outsourcing it to independent testers, so that stories of internal testers being bought off and reporting that they were unable to locate the player will not arise. It is a bit like point-shaving or improper officiating: the stakes are so high that a susceptible tester might make more money by not doing the job than by doing it properly.

While the devil, as always, is in the detail and we'll see how it will work in practice, MLB seems to have finally understood that, concerning doping, it has lost all credibility in the eyes of the public. Therefore, it has agreed to let an unbiased third party that is not connected with the MLB or its players implement the new policy. Depending on how it is implemented, this is a good forward step and one essential for future progress in removing drugs from MLB. We can only hope that the choice will be made in the interests of an effective policy and not one that will fall into the "hear no evil, see no evil, speak no evil" category that has prevailed to date. Analysis of samples will be done by a WADA-accredited laboratory. Key to the process, however, will be the management of test results and the follow up on any positive tests in an open and timely manner. Teams, clean players and the public at large must have confidence that testing and results will be properly dealt with.

This has not been a proud chapter in the history of baseball, although the spin doctors, well paid for their efforts, will try to portray the new agreement as a triumph. They will be helped by the media, who want to continue to report on baseball. But the fact of the matter is that MLB, MLBPA and the media have known of these problems for years but generally chose to ignore them. The Players Association

Pro Sports I: Baseball, Football and Basketball

has had an all-but-free ride on this issue. It is, some say, the strongest union in the world and has no compunction whatsoever about confrontation and throwing its weight around. Its head is Don Fehr, a very confrontational leader of the old steel town ilk. In the media, MLB is a softer target and much easier to hit, especially since it regularly gets out-maneuvered by the Players Association. But MLB has the lion's share of the responsibility for the drug problem in the sport. The drug users are its players, and the MLBPA has consistently fought to prevent drug testing and significant penalties as a deterrent. This incomprehensible political position works against the best interests of the players, who seem to have turned over their rights to union leaders without any critical assessment of what those leaders are doing on their behalf. You would think that the players themselves would be the ones who would be fighting to ensure they did not have to take all that stuff in order to play in MLB. It makes the MLBPA an active accomplice to doping in baseball.

Apologists often say that the home run duels of recent years—Mark McGwire and Sammy Sosa, and then Barry Bonds—saved baseball, whether the balls were hit by juiced-up giants or not. Attendance has soared, they say, fuelled by these exploits. Owners and players are making money. The fans do not seem to care. What could be better? Never mind the message sent to the public and to the admiring youth of the country. Never mind the adoption of the same "who cares about the rules" mentality that led to Enron, WorldCom and scores of other businesses in another portion of the business world. Never mind that players who have followed the rules are put at a disadvantage, both in performance and financially. Never mind that the national sport, played at its highest level, had become a charade. Those who should have been its trustees and champions,

CHAPTER NINE

charged with protecting the integrity of their businesses and the national sport, were complicit. And the latest triumph is deliberately designed as just enough to get Congress off their backs. Not a gram or millimeter more. Some triumph! I sure would not want to be the brand manager for MLB.

The revelations about Bonds and others will be a significant test for MLB and, in particular, for its commissioner, Bud Selig. How he deals with the facts surrounding one of the acknowledged superstars of baseball and how he uses those facts to get an even stricter anti-drug program may be his defining moment. So far, in the spring of 2006, he has announced the appointment of former Senator George Mitchell to investigate the doping allegations. It is unclear what powers Mitchell will have to get information to form the basis for his report, what the scope of his investigation will be and if the Players Association will cooperate and to what degree. Similarly unclear is what Selig will or can do with the eventual findings of the report. My only experience with Mitchell was when he headed up a similar project for the United States Olympic Committee in connection with the Salt Lake City bidding scandal. I confess that I was not very impressed with the quality of his report and the efforts to get at the underlying facts of the involvement of the USOC in the bidding process. It was almost entirely a whitewash operation and a deflection of all blame away from the USOC and anyone in the U.S. in the direction of the IOC. The IOC definitely deserved its share of the blame for the situation, but there were two sides to each infraction, a fact that Mitchell seemed to ignore. One other feature of the MLB investigation is that Mitchell is a director of the Boston Red Sox. I would think that there might be someone, somewhere in America, with the necessary qualities to conduct the investigation but who would have no such obvious conflict of interest.

Pro Sports I: Baseball, Football and Basketball

I may occasionally sound as if I think that MLB is the only professional sport with a drug problem (and I am sure that some connected with baseball may agree), but that, of course, is not true. It's just that no other sport has been as arrogant about first, its denial that a problem actually existed and second, its solution to the problem once its nose was publicly rubbed in the very mess whose existence it had denied. There is no doubt that the other professional leagues have similar drug problems and have been almost as ineffective as MLB in solving them.

THE NATIONAL FOOTBALL LEAGUE

The NFL has the best education program in professional sport regarding drugs. One reason for this may be that the NFL has already gone through and come out the other side of the institutionalized poisonous league-players' association relationships that still exist in other leagues. Both sides seem to understand that the better the NFL brand, the better it is for owners and players alike. But, the questions remain. It is hard to ignore the evidence before your eyes each time you see NFL teams on the field. Maybe it is just lots of mom's oatmeal porridge. Maybe not.

The National Football League (NFL) is far better at its public relations on the doping issue. It claims to have the best anti-drug program in professional sport. The NFL may be right, but if so, it may be damning itself with faint praise. You only have to look at the players in any NFL game to see that there are a quite a few of them who obviously did not get to those sizes and shapes by simply eating mom's porridge at home. How come the much-vaunted NFL program can't seem to catch many of the dopers? How come a disproportionate number of player deaths seem to be in football?

CHAPTER NINE

The NFL's answer to this, when I met with their representatives, as well as the players' representatives, in January 2006, was quite fascinating. I acknowledge that the league is far more adept at massaging these issues than are the others. For one thing, the NFL has little appetite for discussing doping practices of the past, and probably for good reason, given what was going on and the revelations of some of the players of the day. I can still remember the grisly interview given by Lyle Alzado in 1991, not long before his death from cancer, who believed that the disease had been caused by his use of steroids. Other disclosures, including those by Bill Romanowski, who acknowledged extensive steroid use, have made it equally clear that there was a definite drug culture in the game.

Not interested the slightest in discussing what may have gone on in the past, the NHL instead chooses to focus on the problems of today and the changes it says have occurred in recent years. They are today's owners and players and have their collective eye on what lies ahead, regardless of the lessons that are there for the taking in relation to the prior problem and how and why it was ignored. The NFL admits that players are generally bigger than they used to be, but then, they say, so is the population at large. The players are trained to play particular positions that call for more specific body types. The skill sets required of position players allow the teams to recruit accordingly. Today, you don't have to have linemen with the speed and agility to pull and run, as they did years ago; their jobs now are to protect the quarterback or to open holes for the running backs. Now, all they have to be is huge. These days, young players start lifting weights in high school, and their size and strength increase over a period of several years—naturally—not over a matter of months, aided by drugs consumed for

Pro Sports I: Baseball, Football and Basketball

the purpose. Today, unlike in the past, a 300-plus-pound player who retires does not lose fifty or more pounds in the first few months following retirement, but maintains the weight and may even gain more. From this, the NFL concludes—abracadabra—that the players of today are not juiced up to get to the playing weight.

Now, all this may well be absolutely true. I just do not know for sure, although my every instinct screams at me that there is far more here than meets the eye. On the other hand, the NFL has been the most willing of any league to meet with WADA and discuss the details of its programs. They do not necessarily share the results of their tests, but are at least willing to discuss what they do and to look for some guidance in the WADA List for their own list of prohibited substances and methods. Not unexpectedly, the results, if announced, tend to be a combination of steroids and hormones, with the addition of recreational drugs. It clearly has the best education program in professional sport regarding drugs. One reason for this may be that the NFL has already gone through and come out the other side of the institutionalized poisonous league-players' association relationships that still exist in other leagues. Both sides seem to understand that the better the NFL brand, the better it is for owners and players alike.

There are obviously differing interests and objectives in any organization involving owners and players, whether in football or the other professional sports. The owners act together to advance their interests and I see no reason why the players should not do the same, especially since without the collective bargaining position, the players could be picked off one by one in any negotiation. But that does not mean that, within the league, where everyone should be working together to maximize the benefits for all concerned, relations should be confrontational. Not every proposal of

CHAPTER NINE

the owners should be characterized as anti-player and fought, simply because it came from the owners. And *vice versa*. You do not have to die in every single ditch of a negotiation. The other leagues might well learn something from the NFL, at least in organizational behaviour.

We at WADA have agreed to work with the NFL to see how many points of agreement there are between the NFL program and the World Anti-Doping Code. It is clear that we probably will not reach an agreement on penalties for doping offenses that will mirror those in the Code. The NFL says that the average playing life of a player is four years, and that a two-year suspension just will not wash. The league says that its four-game suspensions (now under pressure from the players, who think it's too severe) are sufficient deterrents for other players. They say to have someone sitting out for a quarter of the season, unable to practice with the team, is all but a death sentence for the player. There are too many talented players looking to make their own marks, who will replace suspended players in a heartbeat. They may even do a better job. I confess to being un-persuaded on this. I'm sorry, but a two-game (the players' choice) or even a four-game (the NFL's current position) suspension just is not enough. We are not talking about an offside during a game, but the deliberate use of a prohibited substance ingested for the purpose of getting an advantage over an opponent. The message is all wrong. Where more serious penalties are applied against repeating dopers, the current paid vacation of choice is to send them to the Canadian Football League, which has no testing policy and does not recognize sanctions imposed by the NFL.

As I said, it is all very believable, and I do hope that when we dig down a bit, we will find that what the NFL says is true. But, you could say that I am from Missouri, the "Show Me State." My experience is that if it sounds too good to be true, it usually is.

THE NATIONAL BASKETBALL ASSOCIATION

> *The NBA anti-doping program is not as rigorous as it should be, and it specifically excludes out-of-season testing. In a sport where size does matter, not testing for the use of drugs, such as human growth hormone, during the time when they are most likely to be used is practically an invitation for players to acquire and use them.*

The National Basketball Association (NBA) has had a much more difficult time in coming to terms with an effective anti-doping policy. The most recent collective bargaining process has been particularly difficult, and many issues, including the use of recreational drugs, on-court comportment, anti-social behavior and attitude that were bringing the game into disrepute, needed to be resolved. As a matter of getting the NBA house in order, the priorities had to be aligned and, frankly, the NBA saw doping as farther down the list than most of the other issues. David Stern, a very able and sophisticated commissioner, has had to settle for half a loaf for the time being.

The bargaining process that led to the announcement of the new collective agreement in June 2005 (also under the threat of congressional legislative action) was very difficult and confrontational, and performance-enhancing drugs was only one of several serious issues the association had to consider. In the short run, the NBA sees as its biggest problem the use of social or recreational drugs, not identifying and dealing with performance-enhancing drugs. It is bad for the image of the NBA and for professional basketball in general when players get caught

CHAPTER NINE

using recreational drugs and in other PR nightmares. As a result, the NBA has made recreational drug use a far greater public relations issue than worrying about what the players may do to prepare for competition. The NBA anti-doping program is, therefore, not as rigorous as it should be, and it specifically excludes out-of-season testing. In a sport where size does matter, not testing for the use of drugs, such as human growth hormone, during the time when they are most likely to be used is all but an invitation for players to acquire and use them. It is a huge gap in a program that is put forward as a serious and comprehensive response to an acknowledged problem.

The international basketball federation, known by its French acronym, FIBA, is subject to the WADA Code and wants the NBA to agree to adopt it as well. In the 1992 Games in Barcelona, with the appearance of the first Dream Team, FIBA allowed NBA players to be eligible for Olympic competition. This led to a situation parallel—and equally unsatisfactory—to that in ice hockey (see the next chapter). Once a player in the NBA is selected for his national team, he becomes subject to testing under the World Anti-Doping Code. It is better than nothing, but is annoying and unfair to non-NBA players, who are constantly subject to the Code and liable to testing at any time.

Interestingly enough, as an historical aside, it was not the NBA that was pounding on the Olympic door for admission, although it obviously recognized the value of the astronomical Olympic television coverage for promoting its own business, the recognition of its players and possible increased ratings for subsequent NBA programming. Instead, it was FIBA that recognized that, if there was to be a significant increase in the skill levels in international basketball, the players needed to be exposed to the NBA players, such as Michael Jordan, then the undoubted king of basketball. You could watch all the videos of NBA stars you wanted, but, unless you actually got faked out of your shoes (or worse) on a court with them, you would never have a chance to rise to their level.

So, in the interests of the game at large, FIBA decided to allow the NBA professionals to participate. The first time was in Barcelona in 1992, when the U.S. Dream Team took the floor. Where the gold medal was going was never in doubt. The whole drama of the Olympic competition was to see who would go up against the U.S. in the final. At the start of the gold medal game, the teams lined up and were introduced. Normally, the captains exchange a flag or some other souvenir, while the other players try to look nonchalant or try to stare each other down. This time, the entire opposing team rushed over to have their photographs taken with the NBA stars they admired. Many thought that Olympic basketball would belong to the U.S. for at least thirty years, until others caught up, but by 2000 in Sydney (a mere eight years later), the U.S. was behind at half-time in the final—to France—before eventually getting ahead to win. In Athens in 2004, the U.S. lost the gold medal and only managed to squeak a bronze behind both Argentina and Italy. Run-of-the-mill NBA players are no longer good enough to win in the Olympics. Besides, there are many foreign players starting to play in the NBA, and they take their skills home to their own national teams at Games time. FIBA's strategy for the game has paid off.

WADA will do an audit with the NBA anti-doping program by comparing it with our own program and identifying the differences. FIBA will use its best efforts, along with WADA's, to encourage further progress so that the unfairness of being subject to testing only when the national team may be involved for NBA players, compared to 24/7/365 for all other players, is removed. I see a problem

CHAPTER NINE

similar to that of the NFL regarding penalty periods, but, I hope, most of the other discrepancies can be addressed. With the difficult state of tension between the players and the NBA, there is a practical limit on what can be accomplished in the short run, unless Congress gets active again and threatens legislation. Otherwise, we will have to be patient and see what we can encourage as the next round of negotiations approaches.

So, here we have the three most important professional leagues in the United States, none of which, in my view, have sufficiently vigorous anti-doping programs. One, MLB, has been guilty of institutional denial of a widespread problem and has been dragged, kicking and screaming, to the table in the face of congressional pressure and irrefutable evidence of doping and seems determined to do as little as possible. It will be a real test of the sport to see what is the outcome of the Mitchell investigation and the subsequent action taken by MLB. Next on the scale is the NFL, which has a neater package and better delivery of its message, but woefully weak sanctions and an inclination to consider reducing them even further, combined with a seeming inability to find drug use among its athletes. The NBA, for whatever the reason, has problems that are more crucial to its survival as a business and has, admittedly, put a comprehensive anti-doping problem to one side as it wrestles with comportment and other issues. The whole mix is not one that provides much confidence that the organizations providing the bulk of the sport content experienced by the American public give a damn about the message they send to the public and, above all, its youth regarding the use of performance-enhancing drugs.

10 Pro Sports II: Hockey, Soccer, Golf and Other Sports

In business, money always talks. It is what makes the business world go round. Owners do not want their stars, who are paid huge salaries, to be out of the lineup merely for drug use. They are quite happy to see and encourage a lax policy, while paying lip service to doping-free sport. The owners of the NHL chummily bargained with their players' association for more than thirty years to make sure there were no tests of their players and wrapped themselves in the self-congratulatory mantle of saying that there was no need for a testing program, since there was no drug use in hockey!

With the exception of possibly the stupidest lockout in the history of professional sport that wiped out the 2004–2005 season and led to the removal of the leader of the players' association, Bob Goodenow, the National Hockey League (NHL) operates as a fairly successful business. As an

CHAPTER TEN

organization, it has had the usual reluctance to recognize changes in the game. It has, stubbornly and sadly, refused to expand its playing surfaces to the international size to take into account the increasing size and speed of its players. The result has been a game that is played on surfaces that are too small, and the game has degenerated largely into a clutch-and-grab exercise, albeit now improved to some degree by rule and officiating changes following the lockout. But Canadians and some Americans still love it and are fiercely and uncritically protective of it.

In November 2005, at one of my speaking engagements and interviews on the general subject of doping in sport and the international response to the problem, I was asked whether I thought there was a doping problem in professional hockey. I said that the NHL, like all sports, has a doping problem, since no sport is immune from doping. How many NHL players did I think used performance-enhancing substances? This was not easy to answer because, for the past thirty or more years, the NHL and the NHLPA had collectively agreed to make sure that there was no performance-enhancing drug testing whatsoever of NHL players (although there were some tests for substance abuse). Not a single performance-enhancing drug test. The NHL blandly maintained that there was no need for testing in the NHL because there was no performance-enhancing drug problem in hockey. It is a foolishly circular argument. Don't forget that the people making it are hockey people. They know perfectly well what is going on and that there was and is drug use in the game. They are trying to draw attention away from an embarrassing fact, doubly embarrassing because both sides worked together to ensure that nothing was done about it. I think the opposite approach should be adopted. If there is no drug problem, as the NHL asserts (and this is its assertion), then the NHL should not object to

Pro Sports II: Hockey, Soccer, Golf and Other Sports

a strict testing program to show everyone that its players in fact do not have a doping problem. The NHL should back up what it says: that its game is clean. It would, if true, be so different from the other professional (and amateur) sports that it should be demonstrated.

I couldn't answer the question about how many NHL players I thought used drugs. How could I quote facts and figures when there was, and still is, no data available from the NHL itself? But my best guess was perhaps one-third of NHL players were doping. I based this on information WADA had from former players, coaches, team officials and doctors who treated hockey teams at various levels in the hockey system. If I heard one more time the nonsense that there was no problem in hockey, since none of the substances on the WADA List would be of any assistance to a hockey player, I thought I would throw up. Well, the reaction from the NHL management was entirely predictable and matched MLB's reaction. There was instant denial of any problem and general outrage for daring to suggest that there was. It was particularly convenient for the most foamy mouthed commentators, encouraged by the hockey fraternity, to focus on steroids, as if they were the only "problem" drug. But I deliberately had not limited my comments to steroids, referring to all the drugs—including steroids, stimulants, EPO, human growth hormone—that would lead to a positive test under the World Anti-Doping Code. The NHL demanded proof and threatened to sue me for damaging the integrity of its players. But how could there be any proof since, by collective agreement, there was never any testing whatsoever of its players for performance enhancement? Is it any wonder, then, that there has never been a positive case of doping in the NHL?

The only doping policy that has ever emerged from the NHL was in June 2005. With considerable fanfare, the

CHAPTER TEN

league announced that it and the NHLPA had reached an agreement regarding the use of drugs in hockey. Tests would be required, and sanctions would be imposed on players who tested positive. This sounded like a great leap forward and a long-overdue response to an evident problem, even if the plan was seriously flawed. But it was no coincidence that the announcement followed the 2005 U.S. congressional hearings regarding drug use in professional sport and the threat of anti-doping legislation. As with MLB, the NHL tried to avoid such legislation and get Congress off its case—nothing more. Congress simply did not believe there was no drug problem and considered that the NHL's complete lack of any policy was outrageous. Within days of the NHL's "big announcement," Congress easily identified many of the flaws in the policy and dismissed it as seriously ineffective.

How could you possibly have a meaningful drug-testing program that does not permit out-of-competition testing? That's right, under the NHL's so-called vigorous and rigorous new program, no drug tests are permitted in the off-season (an obvious time for the use of steroids or human growth hormone, for example). And—oops—there will be no tests before or after a game. Nor will there be testing for any stimulants. The NHL policy is deliberately weak. I said at the time that it looked as if the NHL had found an early version of MLB's program and copied it. We asked the NHL to give us a copy of their adopted policy so that we could compare it with WADA's Code. The NHL refused, on the basis that it was a private contract. The league was mad at me, so I couldn't see its policy. At the time of writing, we have still not seen it.

However, congressional attention is notoriously short, and even this weak policy did not result in a single test within the NHL, based on its own announced policy, until

Pro Sports II: Hockey, Soccer, Golf and Other Sports

early 2006. Not one single test. You would think that a policy announced so boldly and ceremoniously in June would be put into effect at the start of the season, in September. There must have been some reason for the delay. Was the NHL's photocopier on the blink for two months? It can't be because the NHL had to educate the players about a no-drug policy, which has been part of the rules for many years. Even those coming up into the NHL or coming from Europe would have already known about drug testing, since that would have been part of their hockey lives for some years. Besides, there was nothing to worry about anyway, since there was no drug use in hockey. Wasn't that the official view of the NHL? Was it possible that some players used the delay to go and get privately tested for whatever they were using? Apparently yes, that's exactly how some of the players used the time. Odd, since there apparently were no drugs in the NHL. Hmmm. And, when there were a couple of positive tests of NHL players (Brian Berard and José Théodore) after the policy was announced, the NHL refused to recognize them as positive, because they were not NHL tests (they related to Olympic participation) and had occurred prior to the time that the NHL eventually began its testing. The two players were cheerfully allowed to continue playing in the NHL.

Late in 2005, I tried to convince NHL Commissioner Gary Bettman that it would be in the best interests of the NHL to work with WADA, voluntarily, to develop a good anti-doping program that would win the approval of Congress and the public. This would be far better than being dragged, despite noisy denials, to the table as a result of legislation. But Bettman insisted that there was no drug problem in the NHL and preferred to give the announced policy (defective as it was) a chance to work.

CHAPTER TEN

I would love to be able to say that WADA is satisfied that there are effective anti-doping programs in place in the NHL as well as the other professional leagues in North America and other parts of the world, so during the Olympics in Turin, I met with Bettman and Ted Saskin, of the NHLPA, to see if we could at least figure out where we agreed and disagreed. But how could we do this, given our respective public positions—mine that there was a drug problem, and theirs, that I am a complete idiot and didn't know what I was talking about? We agreed to discuss the situation on a completely informal basis to see what we could agree on. At any rate, contacts were gradually established, although we have still not seen the NHL anti-doping policy, and the NHL Assistant Commissioner, Bill Daly, joined in supporting Lance Armstrong's pre-2006 Tour de France effort to have me removed as Chairman of WADA.

Prior to 2006, NHL players only had to take tests for performance-enhancing drugs if they participated in the Olympic Games and world championships. The International Ice Hockey Federation (IIHF) has an out-of-competition and in-competition testing program, and all athletes involved became subject to the testing. The NHL players did not want to be tested by their national authorities, and I always wondered why not. Perhaps they were concerned that they might not have been forgiving enough, or perhaps they thought that it might lead to multiple tests from different national agencies every time they happened to be in another country. After much negotiation, the NHL players finally agreed to WADA-organized tests. But all this sounds much better than it really is. They did not need to be tested until they were selected or declared themselves willing to be selected for international competition. This means that for about three-and-a-half years out of the four between Olympic Games,

Pro Sports II: Hockey, Soccer, Golf and Other Sports

there is no testing, and the benefits of any doping activity can be carried forward into the Olympic competition, giving them an obvious advantage over non-NHL players who are subject to regular testing. The possibility of testing would occur more often if the players were taking part in the annual world championships.

In an effort to show that there is no drug problem in the NHL, the league points out that there have been very few, if any, positive results from such tests. However, it fails to note that players have plenty of time to prepare themselves to be drug-free for the pre-Olympic testing program. Of course, the NHL never mentions the embarrassingly small number of tests that have actually been performed—as well as what is *not* tested for.

There are still sports writers who do not get it. During the Turin Winter Games, one Canadian expert actually wrote (and as Dave Barry used to say, I am not making this up) that if the NHL said there was no drug testing because there was no need for it, then there was obviously no problem. What a sophisticated and penetrating conclusion! I say that if there is no doping problem in the NHL, then prove it to the public that you have concretely determined this. There should be no problem with having a strict testing program and imposing tough penalties. If there is no problem, there should be no problem. As said many times before, doping is very seldom accidental. The Code allows for reduced sanctions for relatively minor doping infractions and if it's not really the athlete's fault. The possibility of genuine mistakes can be built into the process. The same columnist also criticized my suggestion that, for decades, the NHL had negotiated drug testing out of its collective bargaining agreements. This fool Pound, he implied, has it all wrong. It was not the NHL that wanted there to be no tests, but the NHL Players' Association! Sounds like a two-minute course

CHAPTER TEN

on the notion of contracts might be helpful. But perhaps I give him too much credit. He didn't speculate as to why the NHLPA would have taken such a strenuous position against having tests, especially if there were no drug problem in the first place. Hmmmm...

The most recent development was the announcement in June 2006 that the NHL had conducted some 1,400 tests and that they were all negative. This was evidence that I had been all wrong and that, as the NHL had always maintained, there was no drug problem in hockey. I could hardly believe my ears. After several months of preparing for tests, with continual notice to the players that they were coming, the NHL tested for steroids and not, for example, stimulants, during the season only, and had the chutzpah to conclude that there was no drug problem in hockey! If it were not so serious, it would be laughable.

There will be no hope for hockey until its leaders and players step up to the recognition of the problem. It looks as if they will need help to do so.

SOCCER: THE FIFA FACTOR

> *FIFA, the international federation governing soccer, has tried to have it both ways. Even though it does not allow its best players to compete in the Olympics, the Olympics are still an important showcase for soccer. It would be dreadful for its image if the International Olympic Committee excluded soccer because FIFA refused to adopt WADA's anti-doping rules.*

Soccer is by far the single most popular sport in the world, played in virtually every country and, depending on the traditions in each country, by school-aged children to the multimillionaire professionals. The World Cup, held

Pro Sports II: Hockey, Soccer, Golf and Other Sports

every four years, draws television audiences that rival the Olympic audiences, and some countries are so transfixed by the event that they virtually close down while the World Cup games are played. The Fédération Internationale de Football Association (FIFA), the international federation governing soccer, earns hundreds of millions of dollars per year and is immensely powerful.

With this power comes a certain disdain for being part of any consensus within the sport world. It does not, for example, permit its best players to take part in the Olympic Games, relegating the Olympic tournament to little more than a junior world championship because of the age limits, under twenty-three, on the players in the Olympics. Because of the universality of the sport, the Olympic authorities have meekly accepted the decree of FIFA. Fortunately for the Olympics, no other sport on the Olympic program is strong enough to thumb its nose at the idea that the Olympics should be available to the best players in the world. The only one that comes close is tennis, where all the best players are eligible, even though many of them, independent contractors as they are, do not bother to show up.

Not surprisingly, FIFA's attitude is reflected in the fight against doping in sport. FIFA continues to chant the mantra that there is no doping problem in soccer, even after it has become ridiculous. It astonishes me how sport leaders (and not just in soccer) can persist with such positions and utter them in public with a straight face.

Since the adoption of the Code by WADA in 2003, all Olympic sports must adopt and apply the Code in order for the sport to remain on the Olympic program. Since then, FIFA has tried to have it both ways. Even though it does not allow its best players to compete, the Olympics are still an important showcase for soccer. It would be dreadful for

CHAPTER TEN

its image if the International Olympic Committee excluded soccer because FIFA refused to adopt WADA's anti-doping rules. There was much huffing and puffing within the corridors of FIFA as reason after reason was trotted out for either not adopting the Code or for making exceptions applicable to FIFA.

As the deadline for adoption of the Code prior to the Games in Athens in 2004 approached, the hard-liners in FIFA seemed to have traction, and it appeared as if the association might not be willing to adopt the Code at its Congress in Paris in June 2004. I had been invited, as president of WADA, to attend the Congress, but I told FIFA President Joseph Blatter that I was not willing to participate unless he could assure me that the Congress would adopt the Code. We went through the various issues that had been raised, and I tried to show how each of these had already been addressed. He was not sure his executive committee would understand, so I offered to go back to my Paris hotel and write out, verbatim, what I would be willing to say to his Congress. It took a couple of hours (I type slowly), but I e-mailed it to him the same afternoon. He called back to say that, if I said exactly what I had written, he thought the Congress would approve. I told him to give a copy of my draft to his executive committee so they could follow it word by word. Following my intervention the next day, the Congress unanimously adopted the Code.

I hoped that this would be the end of the matter, but dealing with FIFA turned out to be more complicated. Adopting the Code was one thing, but changing the internal FIFA rules to comply with the Code was yet another. There didn't seem to be too much difficulty with the medical rules, but the disciplinary rules proved to be more problematic. FIFA has a system for dealing with doping infractions that it describes as "individual case management." It wants to

Pro Sports II: Hockey, Soccer, Golf and Other Sports

treat each case separately. I could not agree more—every case is an individual case—and that is precisely what happens under the Code, where the sanctions can vary from a warning to two years, depending on the substance used and the degree of fault surrounding the use. We have done our best to convince FIFA that this is the same as individual case management, but to no avail. I think the real reason is that FIFA wanted to be free to impose sanctions of less than two years, the default sanction under the Code, even when an athlete failed to establish that there was no significant fault on his part.

We jockeyed back and forth, without success, for a year or so to see if we could reach an agreement on suitable wording for its disciplinary rules. Finally, in May 2005, WADA issued a preliminary finding that FIFA was not complying with the World Anti-Doping Code, which would mean that soccer would not be allowed in the Olympics, and that there would be difficulties for the 2006 World Cup because governments also insist that the Code rules be applied. Because there was another FIFA Congress coming up in September 2005, I suggested that WADA delay official notification of the finding in order to give FIFA one last chance to change its rules. Probably for the tenth time, we offered to work with them to find the right language, but got no response.

FIFA then made some changes and sent them to us. It announced that it was now compliant with the Code. Actually, the way FIFA likes to position it is that WADA is now FIFA-compliant! Aren't egos wonderful?

It was obvious to us that FIFA was still far from being compliant. However, instead of getting into yet another endless "my lawyer is bigger than your lawyer" discussion, we decided to short-circuit the process and to request an advisory opinion from CAS. For many reasons, it was

CHAPTER TEN

important that there be no separate and lesser rules for FIFA, as this would only encourage other federations to ask for special treatment as well. We needed to have one set of harmonized rules for everyone. The CAS panel found, as we expected, that FIFA was non-compliant in several significant respects, and FIFA agreed to make the changes necessary prior to the 2006 World Cup in Germany. It has reluctantly done so, but made sure that the changes only came into effect following the World Cup. The pressure on FIFA was that if it failed to make the changes, then WADA would have persisted with making final our preliminary determination of non-compliance, which would have created great difficulties for Germany as host of the 2006 World Cup (and a country that had approved the 2005 UNESCO Convention) and for the IOC, which would have had to consider what the implications would be for the 2008 Olympics in Beijing.

In the end, whatever the CAS decision might have been, it was a win-win scenario of WADA and a lose-lose situation for FIFA. We won, and FIFA had to change its rules. If, however, CAS had concluded that the FIFA rules as drafted were effectively the same as the Code rules, I was ready to apply the Code rules regarding sanctions, including our right to appeal against any FIFA doping decisions, and leave FIFA with the uphill argument that its rules, despite the CAS opinion, were nevertheless different from the Code, and different from what it had already argued in the CAS proceedings.

The bottom line, however, is that the most important sport in the world is now applying the same anti-doping rules as the other sports. This is an excellent message for sport in general and I hope we can work more cooperatively in future with FIFA and take advantage of its vast network of international sports, medical and educational resources.

Pro Sports II: Hockey, Soccer, Golf and Other Sports

PROFESSIONAL GOLF: THE PGA

Golf is possibly the sport that has the least problems with drugs. However, having said that, it is becoming increasingly obvious that the shapes of some of the professional golfers have begun to change to leaner, stronger physiques, noticeably different from the blobby appearance of many of the longer-term golfers, and not all the difference in the length off the tee is the result of advances in ball and club technology. This adds a new dimension to the general knowledge that beta blockers were used to control the basic tremor that everyone has but which tends to increase with age and can have a significant effect on putting. There is no reason to believe that other performance-enhancing drugs are unknown to golfers. I have tried, so far without success, to persuade the PGA commissioner, Tim Finchem, to take a leadership role among professional sports by adopting a meaningful anti-doping policy and implementing it. Golfers are generally self-policing and very honest during their play, to a degree unmatched in almost any other sport. So, I thought it would be an additional chevron of the integrity of the game of golf to say, "We do not think there is a problem, but we are willing to be tested in order to demonstrate this to the public." It is one thing to declare yourself to be without sin, but better still to have some independent proof of the claim, especially when some of your best players, like Nick Price and Greg Norman, have publicly stated that there is, in fact, a drug problem in the PGA.

There is no doubt that the physical appearances of many professional golfers—both men and women—are different from even a few years ago, and there are more and more golfers pumping iron in the gyms. I do hope that golfers do not fall back on the same lame excuse as the baseball players—that it's hand-eye coordination that generates the

CHAPTER TEN

power, and that bulging muscles are irrelevant. However, Finchem does not want golf to be tainted by association with the other sports that are replete with drugs. He thinks it would be bad for golf if the public were to associate golfers with athletes in the other sports where there are known to be doping problems. To date, I have not been able to convince him that, on the contrary, he would do more for his sport by leading rather than following the others. There is no doubt that, one way or another, professional golf—both men's and women's—will have to implement an anti-drug program—eventually. It is only a matter of time before details of drug use will become known.

OTHER PROFESSIONAL SPORTS

We have made ongoing efforts to persuade other sports to come on board and have enjoyed some success. Tennis, through the Association of Tennis Players (ATP), has after much hesitation agreed to ally itself with the International Tennis Federation (ITF) and to apply the World Anti-Doping Code, and I hope that discussions with the Women's Tennis Association (WTA) will also bring the women players onside in future. Cricket, perhaps smarting from the disclosures of cheating on the field of play, has agreed to adopt the Code, as has rugby. Horse racing has been concerned for years about drug use in the sport, made all the more complicated by the fact that horses cannot communicate sufficiently and by the uncertain line between therapy and doping. I do not know to what degree there may be rigorous testing of jockeys, who may find stimulants to be helpful to maintain alertness or diuretics to "make weight." Professional boxing has different rules from those applicable to Olympic boxing, but has been known to find the occasional fighter to have tested positive.

Pro Sports II: Hockey, Soccer, Golf and Other Sports

ARE PROFESSIONAL SPORTS REAL OR NOT?

The public is entitled to the genuine article, not some knock-off concocted by the players and the owners of the teams as some generic Brand X. If they are not willing to do it on their own, someone should force them to do it. Perhaps it is time to consider external regulation, in the way gambling and racing are regulated by state authorities.

The time is coming when the public, the owners, the players and, perhaps, governments will have to decide where the real values of professional sport lie. The public and government may have to decide whether self-regulation produces the best results. If professional sport degenerates into pure entertainment and not genuine competition, that's one thing. If, on the other hand, it holds itself out as real competition, where outcomes are not determined in advance, with applicable rules, and invites the public to buy into that model, it will need to ensure that the rules are enforced in order to guarantee the integrity of the competition. The public is entitled to the genuine article, not some knock-off concocted by the players and the owners of the teams as some generic Brand X. If they are not willing to do it on their own, someone should force them to do it. Perhaps it is time to consider external regulation, in the way gambling and racing are regulated by state authorities.

I must say that I have not made up my mind as to the best solution. The U.S. Congress acts through legislation, its default solution to almost any issue that comes before it. The problem with some legislation, especially if it is enacted quickly and emotionally, is that it risks being too extreme. Quite simply, if too extreme, it will end up not being enforced. One can only hope that the league leaders

CHAPTER TEN

and players are not too short-sighted to recognize the risk and not so foolish as to ignore it. Legislating mandatory drug tests all the way down to high school sports may well be too heavy-handed and both difficult and expensive to implement and monitor. What would be ideal would be to persuade those involved in sport to acknowledge that the World Anti-Doping Code deals with the problems in a suitable manner and that the use of the Court of Arbitration for Sport will avoid costly and conflicting results before the regular courts, a recourse that would be available to them, should they choose to use it. This would allow them to adopt those rules as part of their own, without the need for federal legislation. I much prefer to see sport govern itself, rather than have unilateral government interference in its operations. This is quite different from the partnership we have established through WADA, in which we work cooperatively to find solutions to problems in which each side, sport and government, makes the appropriate contributions. In some cases, sport leads the issue, and in others it is the governments that take the lead. But, if sport is unwilling to take its responsibilities seriously, then it will have to live with the results, however unappetizing and ponderous government intervention may be.

The best solution is one that provides for equal treatment of all athletes and all sports—both amateur and professional. I can see no reason why professional sports should have different rules for performance-enhancing drugs from amateur sports in the Olympics. Money, as far as I am concerned, is not a relevant justification for different rules. Some rich athletes feel that they make far too much money to be bothered with the rules against drug use. But that is certainly not a reason to allow lax enforcement of the rules. I regularly ask professional sports people to name the substances or procedures identified in the WADA List

Pro Sports II: Hockey, Soccer, Golf and Other Sports

that the leagues believe their players should be allowed to use or do. There is never a satisfactory answer—because there is no satisfactory answer.

Many like to blame money as the root of all evil in sport. There is no question that money influences some behavior, but there was cheating in sport long before there was any money in it. In the professional sports, I have long suspected that owners of teams have little, if any, interest in serious sanctions for drug use by their players. After all, why would an owner have any interest in seeing a player whose rights may have been acquired for millions of dollars sitting on the sidelines for two years for a nuisance drug use suspension. The owners pay good—in many cases, excessive—money to their athletes, and they want value for that money, in every game of every season. They simply do not much care what the athletes do to prepare themselves for those games. The owners may wrap themselves in sanctimonious statements about fair play, the health of their athletes and the good of the game, but their actions (or lack of them) speak so much louder than their words. Sadly, much the same criticism can be laid at the doorstep of some athletes, who are willing to do whatever they have to do to keep their income stream going, especially late in their careers. The enormous changes in Barry Bonds occurred in what might otherwise have been the twilight of his career.

The whole question of professional sport and drug use within it is both simpler and more complicated than it may appear at first glance. It is simpler, because if there were a resolve to keep the sport clean and to have zero tolerance, the leagues could easily institute a system of education and sanctions that would have a deterrent effect. There is nothing magic about such a program, and actions to enforce it would be relatively easy to implement. The question is more difficult because we are not in a new position to start

CHAPTER TEN

with clean canvas in front of us. Structures and institutions have been built up over a period of many years and parties have negotiated rights and advantages that they will be unwilling to give up. The situation is not one that calls for the design of a brand new system, but one that needs to be changed. As everyone knows, if you want to be unpopular, try to change something. I think that the major effort should go into trying to get all sides of the professional sport world to understand that it would be better for them to have drug-free sport—better for the sport, better for the public, better for the youth of the world. Sport should be a genuine integration in society, not one tainted by drug use.

Drug Cartels and Drug Pushers in the Wide World of Sport

The performance-enhancing drug business has become extremely profitable. Interpol reports that, financially, steroids and related drugs exceed marijuana, cocaine and heroin combined. In fact, organized crime most likely controls some sections of this lucrative and prohibited market. Doping in sport has become a new venture for drug cartels, drug dealers and drug pushers.

Where do all the performance-enhancing drugs come from? Drugs in sport are not confined to the end users, the athletes. Someone has to produce them. Someone has to distribute them. Someone has to buy them. And someone has to administer them. Doping in sport has created a ripple effect and a full food chain, a problem that needs attention.

CHAPTER ELEVEN

PRODUCTION—IT'S ALL ABOUT THE MONEY

About eighty percent of EPO produced by the pharmaceutical companies is not used for therapeutic purposes, but for doping in sport. In 2004, there were US$11.8 billion sales of EPO worldwide—some 236 million doses. Only about $1.5 billion was for therapeutic use. Yet the pharmaceutical companies that manufacture the drug have been quite blasé. It's not surprising, since they are in the business of making money—big money.

Let's start with the production. Many of the substances used for cheating in sport started off as products that had a therapeutic purpose. That is why they were invented and patented in the first place. Erythropoietin (EPO) is a perfect example. It is produced in the kidneys and stimulates bone marrow to release more oxygen-carrying red blood cells. This is particularly important in assisting anaemic patients with chronic kidney failure or cancer patients undergoing chemo- or radiotherapy to maintain a normal level of red blood cells. Some EPO is produced naturally, but there is also a manufactured version that almost entirely reproduces natural EPO. It is now possible to distinguish between the two, so we can identify whether EPO has been administered from an external source. But, in treating illness, the closer you can get to the natural EPO, the better for the patient, and there is ongoing research to make the artificial EPO even closer to the real thing. This will make it even more difficult for it to be detected. At the moment, it is not possible to insert "markers" like codes that would identify the source of the artificial EPO so that detection can be easier. Any change, even the insertion of the marker, would mean that the product would have to be resubmitted to the FDA or other regulators. That could take years and cost a fortune. Also, the whole idea (for therapeutic purposes) was to make the artificial product as close to natural as possible, and the markers would defeat that purpose. From the perspective of the pharmaceutical industry, I can understand these as legitimate concerns.

Those inclined to cheat in sport are always on the lookout for new ways to do so, especially if the new product is undetectable in the tests that have been developed to date. It does not take a rocket scientist to figure out that a substance that increases the oxygen-carrying capacity of the blood can boost performance significantly. So, EPO became a drug of choice for many athletes, initially in duration events, such as cross-country skiing, cycling and distance running. In recent years, this has spread to other sports and events not generally noted for endurance. These days, even sprinters use EPO.

A recent study by the Belgian government indicates that about eighty percent of the EPO produced is not used for treating illness, but for doping in sport. Furthermore, international organizations such as Interpol and the World Health Organization have taken a look at the situation concerning doping drugs. They both concluded that there is massive overproduction of these drugs that cannot be accounted for on a therapeutic basis. According to official world sales figures in 2004, there were US$11.8 billion sales of EPO (produced by Amgen, Johnson & Johnson, Roche, Kirin, Sankyo)—some 236 million doses. With 300,000 known patients requiring treatment, this accounted for only approximately $1.5 billion. Doing the math, this meant that for each patient requiring EPO, there were 6.8 other customers.

Growth hormone production is much the same story. The global sales were $1.8 billion—some 36 million doses. It is used to help kids with stunted growth to grow, but given the fact that there are only 32,000 pediatric patients, this would

CHAPTER ELEVEN

account for $320 million. That means that for every patient requiring treatment, there were 4.6 other consumers.

Bear in mind that these are official figures based on financial reporting. They do not reflect knock-off or illicit sales that are unreported. It is relatively easy to determine the sales from public or officially reporting companies, but almost impossible when the drugs are knock-offs of patented drugs or generic drugs that are made by anyone once the patent protection period has expired. Official figures are not available regarding steroids. There is no international agency that appears capable of dealing with the issue. The World Health Organization has tried to regulate conscious overproduction of drugs that have doping potential and are a significant portion of the illicit traffic.

These astonishing figures regarding overproduction have not resulted in any kind of reaction from the pharmaceutical industry that manufactures the drugs. I am not surprised, since the industry sells and profits from them. They are in the business of making money—big money. Since the amount of EPO used as a therapeutic drug does not change dramatically year over year, how does the pharmaceutical industry account for the five-fold increase in its sales in 2004? Manna from heaven?

For example, back in 1998, did the industry wonder where the EPO was obtained when the French police discovered industrial quantities of the drug in the possession of the Festina team in the Tour de France? A year or so later, Edita Rumsas, the wife of Lithuanian rider Raimondas Rumsas, was arrested by the same police with a car full of doping substances—thirty-seven different ones, including EPO, testosterone, human growth hormone and anabolic steroids. France has been somewhat ahead of the curve in having strong legislation and a will to enforce it. It did not particularly matter whether there was a sport element to

Drug Cartels and Drug Pushers in the Wide World of Sport

the possession of such drugs, although it was not difficult to expect that a bit of observation would likely lead to locating the persons in possession of drugs used in sport.

The police have not disclosed the sources of the supplies, whether from legitimate or illicit manufacturers, or whether they have been able to trace the drugs back to their source. In many cases there are reports of such drugs being stolen from warehouses, which suggests that organized crime may also be involved in the distribution of the drugs. These factors increase the difficulties of getting convictions at the supply end of the chain, while it is quite easy when catching those in possession. Rumsas let his wife remain in custody for several weeks while he stayed out of the country, beyond the reach of the French police. In the end, he was caught doping in the 2003 Giro d'Italia and suspended. In 2005, the French charged him with importing prohibited drugs and he was convicted. Sadly, these statistics have not led to any significant internal reviews within the industry.

It seems that the pharmaceutical industry is complicit in the spread of doping in sport, especially because of the dramatic increase in production of drugs such as EPO. There doesn't seem to be any other explanation. Both drug companies and regulators are simply not doing their jobs. Does this remind you of the National Rifle Association's saying that guns do not kill people—people kill people?

I remember, back in 1998, when I was working on the concept of the independent international anti-doping agency that became WADA, I thought that a representative of the pharmaceutical industry could be of enormous assistance. We had scheduled a world conference on doping in sport in Lausanne in early February 1999. I discovered that there was an international association of pharmaceutical companies headquartered just down the highway from Lausanne, in Geneva. I invited the association to participate in the

CHAPTER ELEVEN

conference and explained the objectives, but I was advised that, unfortunately, the association had no budget for such purpose and that it would not attend. The train fare was only about twenty Swiss francs, less than $20. Maybe I should have offered to pay this non-budgeted expenditure, about the price of toast and coffee in Geneva. That was an early indication of the degree of help we might expect from the pharmaceutical industry. And almost ten years later, with the exception of some discreet help from a couple of companies on one-off projects, nothing has changed in this respect.

Later on, once WADA was up and running, I had the idea (insanely naive, as it turned out), that we might be able to get the leading international pharmaceutical companies to support the idea of a research fund to help finance investigation into doping substances and methods, so that we could better detect their use by athletes. I thought that, if we could get, say, the five largest companies to lead the way with a commitment of $5 million a year for five years, we could then ask fifty smaller companies to commit $200,000 a year for the same five years. This would give us $175 million for research purposes. We would offer to share the results of the research with all contributing companies and publish the scientific findings. The amount of money involved was small for an industry of that size, but the outcome would be quite significant for WADA. It seemed like such a sensible idea, and I thought the industry would jump at the chance to help the fight against the improper use of its products (great public relations, as a bonus!) and also to benefit from some common research. I wrote a letter to the chairman of Pfizer Inc., as I thought he would be interested in the idea. The company was a natural industry leader, having helped fund, for a number of years, a very prestigious prize for sport medicine. It seemed like a natural avenue of approach.

Drug Cartels and Drug Pushers in the Wide World of Sport

Wrong! There was no interest whatsoever—not the slightest. At a recent invitation of the British sports minister, Richard Caborn, I met with representatives of the pharmaceutical industry, and the reception of the idea was exactly the same. Instead of looking at it as a positive public relations strategy (along with the benefits of all the research), they thought that it would make it look as if they had been complicit in the improper use of their products. They also claimed that it was not *their* products that were in play, but those for which the patents had expired and that were being manufactured by generic drug companies. The companies with proprietary information regarding doping substances would not touch the idea of official collaboration with WADA with the proverbial barge pole, whether on a company-by-company or industry basis. The closest we could get them to any kind of cooperation was that they might be willing to share some of their research on the properties of some of their products. If I had it to do over again—and I might—I think I would go directly to their marketing or public relations departments and convince them that such a strategy would have a very positive effect on their image as a caring corporate citizen that supports drug-free sport and aims to protect young athletes against the pressures and dangers of using performance-enhancing drugs. God knows they need help in the image department, and this strategy would certainly help. They just might pay attention.

To some degree the pharma companies may have a point. Aside from the Belgian findings noted above, a good deal of the illegal traffic in drugs used for performance enhancement seems to be coming from generic manufacturers in India, China and elsewhere. The international controls needed to capture the products as they cross borders have not been developed. Law enforcement agencies have tended to focus on narcotics and social drugs, rather than on steroids and other sports drugs. Domestically, neither India nor China has shown much inclination to toughen their own controls regarding production of these substances. With the increasing attention being given by governments to doping in sport, it may be possible for the sports movement to encourage stricter enforcement.

DISTRIBUTION—DRUG PUSHERS

> *If a doctor is caught pushing performance-enhancing drugs, he won't be able to be a team physician for five years. So what! He probably couldn't care less. But suspending a doctor's right to practice medicine for a period of time and publicly announcing it would be meaningful. It would make a doctor think twice about supplying dope to athletes.*

In the meantime, since the pharmaceutical industry was washing its hands of the entire issue, we needed to look elsewhere. One obvious place was the governments, which have the power to regulate substances by either forbidding their use or controlling them. Obviously, we do not want to make it difficult for doctors and their patients to have access to these substances for legitimate treatments. Our intention is to try to persuade others to not use the substances for performance enhancement. If we are unsuccessful, then we would want to detect the use and penalize the users and those who help them cheat. Both these things can be achieved if the products are controlled by requiring a prescription from a licensed medical practitioner before the product can be obtained. Of course, there are doctors who are willing to prescribe virtually anything their patients ask for.

Governments can further assist here by insisting that medical professionals give prescriptions solely for genuine medical needs and then only in the amounts consistent with such needs. For example, several athletes have obtained TUEs for certain substances, for genuine medical conditions, but when tested the athletes had ten or twenty times the prescribed levels of the substances in their systems. The professional bodies that regulate the practice of medicine must, then, make sure that these standards are followed and discipline their members who do not comply. It is not enough to confine these rules to physicians who specialize in sports medicine. Penalizing someone only in the sports context means nothing. So what if the doctor cannot be a team physician for five years? He or she probably couldn't care less. What's the big deal of losing the opportunity to provide free services to an Olympic team once every four years? It has to become a code of conduct for the profession as a whole in order to become meaningful. Suspending a doctor's right to practice medicine for a period of time and publicly announcing such a sanction would do it.

Records of prescriptions for prohibited or regulated substances should be regularly audited, along with records of purchasers. Doctors should have an obligation to know their patients and to be sure that athletes under their care are not prescribed prohibited substances unless they are for therapeutic use only and then in appropriate quantities only. Athletes have been known to shop around, to get multiple prescriptions and to find doctors who will prescribe the substances they want. Failure to keep adequate records and issuing improper prescriptions should be considered professional misconduct and dealt with accordingly. To date, virtually nothing has been done about this issue. And that is in the developed countries. In the developing world, the situation is far less controlled because the regulatory mechanisms simply do not exist.

It may be surprising to learn that many of the products that are used in doping in sports are also used in veterinary

CHAPTER ELEVEN

practice, where the regulatory framework is not always as refined as it is for human medicine. Drugs such as testosterone and anabolic steroids have been used for years for "bulking up" beef cattle, so why not also for beefing up athletes who can benefit from muscle bulk and strength? It seems to be much easier to get prohibited substances through your friendly neighborhood vet, so that is the route that many take.

The sports movement has adopted its own rules against trafficking in prohibited substances, and it has the right to punish anyone involved in trafficking, but the overwhelming tendency has been to confine the penalties to the athletes who test positive, not to the enablers—the drug pushers. This is largely because of the difficulty in getting evidence. This is something that we would like to change. The pushers are at least as guilty as the users. But there is almost nothing the sports movement can do to stop the trafficking done nationally and internationally outside the established sports structures. This is a matter for governments and international organizations, such as Interpol, as well as national police forces. Once again, many governments, agencies and the police tend to focus on the "hard" drugs, such as heroin, cocaine and, to a lesser degree in some countries, marijuana. They are not very worried about sports drugs, and, in many cases, they are not even aware of the problem.

If Interpol is active in trying to repress illicit international trafficking in performance-enhancing drugs, it does not appear in its annual reports. The U.S. Drug Enforcement Administration (DEA) has examined the problem of doping drugs, but references to them in annual reports is only sporadic, suggesting that there are not many concrete actions in the field, undoubtedly because the focus on drugs has tended to be on the so-called recreational drugs

Drug Cartels and Drug Pushers in the Wide World of Sport

like marijuana, hash, cocaine and heroin. However, they have been aware for some time that illicit trafficking in performance-enhancing drugs was becoming increasingly serious. In December 1993, at an international conference on abuse and trafficking of anabolic steroids (only one of the many doping products), the DEA reported that between 1991 and 1993, U.S. authorities seized more than six million doses of performance-enhancing substances. The primary sources for steroids entering the U.S. were Eastern Europe and South America. Many of the traffickers were involved with drugs other than steroids, especially cocaine, and they were well organized at the highest level. This is going to take a much closer cooperation than has ever existed in the past between the sports and public authorities, and WADA will prove to be the coordinating organization, through its monitoring of the World Anti-Doping Code and by working with the governments for the same objective, using the framework of the 2005 UNESCO Convention Against Doping in Sport. Governments need to know from sport what is going on, where to look, what to look for and perhaps even whom to look for. Some of this will be new ground for most government enforcement agencies, and they will benefit from the experience that sport has gained over the past few years.

Governments were urged by Interpol, WADA and many sport organizations to strengthen controls over anabolic agents to curb their diversion into illicit traffic, as well as to identify manufacturers and quantities produced, imported and exported. International organizations such as WHO were similarly encouraged to get involved to obtain the active cooperation of the pharmaceutical industry in the fight against sports doping. Very few of the countries attending the conference did anything. No one seemed willing to spearhead the creation of an international body capable of dealing

CHAPTER ELEVEN

with the issue. I am sure that in many of the less-developed countries, sport is a matter of very low priority and that they have neither the interest nor the resources necessary to sink teeth into fighting doping. It would not surprise me greatly if there were not some political pressures in countries where the drugs are made through which they encourage non-action. If there is no overwhelming political consensus for coordinated international action, there is unlikely to be any progress, since international problems require international solutions. WADA is committed to pursuing this joint agenda and will be in a better position to do so once the UNESCO Convention comes into formal effect following ratification by the member states.

Countries like France and Italy have made possession of and trafficking in certain substances a criminal offense. Italy has successfully prosecuted and convicted a well-known sports doctor, Michele Ferrari, for his role in assisting athletes to dope, although an appeal court overturned the conviction, partly on the basis of a statute of limitations. Another doctor, Riccardo Agricola, treated the Juventus team that won the European soccer championships in 1994–1998. During his trial, the judge apparently reached the conclusion that some or all of that team had been doped, but that, in the prosecution, there was only one defendant in front of him. This case is still under appeal. Juventus is now in the news again with allegations of manipulating soccer officials, and the police are investigating the team, as well as the whole structure of football in Italy. Who says corruption can be confined to particular silos? The prosecutions in the Balco case in the United States (discussed elsewhere in this book) are another case in point. Governments can act in this field if they wish, and their actions will deter other possible offenders. It's one thing to be embarrassed by the sports media, but it's quite another to know that you could go to jail.

DISTRIBUTION: ORGANIZED CRIME

> *Where activities are not effectively regulated and profits are large, it is certain that organized crime will not be far behind. Available evidence suggests that in many countries, organized crime is intimately involved in the traffic of doping products.*

In January 2005, Russian police uncovered and seized a clandestine plant that was producing anabolic steroids. The plant was not large, but it was capable of producing approximately 150 million doses per year. The single machine used for the purpose had been manufactured in Ukraine, which suggests a much higher production capacity in that country. The South Africa Border Police seized 26,500 pounds of steroid tablets in 2003–2004. Exports from China and India are on the rise. The Italian government has identified criminal involvement in many aspects of illicit traffic in Italy, some for use in Italy and some coming into Italy from outside for trans-shipment. During 2005, Russian organized crime sold steroids to the Arabian Gulf countries, through Kuwait, and these steroids have been sold directly by Russians and local Arabs to, among others, American soldiers in Iraq.

In society, it now appears that many of the same people who supply narcotics—organized crime—are also supplying doping products. If the authorities have been less than successful in stemming the trade in narcotics, the gap is even greater where the laws are weak.

WHO'S BUYING THESE DRUGS?

> *Many sports figures use the banned substances and these stars have enormous influence on young people. They have made it seem cool to use drugs for purely narcissistic*

CHAPTER ELEVEN

reasons. High school girls, as young as grade niners, are using steroids to tone their bodies.

Apart from athletes, it is interesting to observe that the military and police are major users of steroids and doping substances, both for improved performance and appearance. In war or military situations, or anywhere that extreme vigilance is combined with performance criteria, there seems to be little hesitation in using doping methods. Performance is what matters, not how it is achieved. The military is a major user of doping products. This practice goes back at least to the Assassins, members of the fanatical Nizari branch of the Ismaili Muslims, who were active at the time of the Crusades and whose name is derived from the Arabic word for hashish-eater, referring to a substance they apparently used before their missions. The Germans supplied their troops during World War II with testosterone to make them more aggressive. Allied pilots during the same war used stimulants before their raids and soporifics later to get to sleep. Benzedrine was in regular use as a stimulant. There are reports of stimulants now in use that enable pilots and others on missions in Iraq and Afghanistan to remain alert and functioning for forty-eight or more hours at a time. Where there are no rules, there are no rules.

Recently, Interpol and others have concluded that the economic value of the so-called illegal steroid market now exceeds the combined economic value of the marijuana, cocaine and heroin markets, a figure measured in the billions of dollars each year. Not all of this use occurs within organized sport, which is good on the one hand and bad on the other. It is good because one would hate to think that so many billions of dollars are devoted to people trying to cheat their way to winning in sports. It is bad because, to a large degree, the behavior of sports figures, their evident

Drug Cartels and Drug Pushers in the Wide World of Sport

use of the substances and the enormous influence they have on young people have made it seem cool to use drugs for purely narcissistic reasons. High school girls, as young as grade niners, are using steroids to tone their bodies. Gymnasiums are full of peddlers willing to provide steroids. Your kids probably have "friends" willing to supply anything they want. The Internet is full of offers to anyone who can provide money or a credit card number, along with the means to beat any tests to which you might be subject. Keep an eye on them, because these drugs can be addictive and can lead to many problems for teenagers, including depression and death. We have to keep pushing legislators to do their jobs. This will eventually force governments to act on what will become a public health problem—just as U.S. Congress has begun to tighten the screws on the professional sports leagues.

Entrenched financial interests, whether over or under the legal table, are not going to do anything to prevent or reduce the traffic in performance-enhancing drugs on their own initiative. They are making good money. That is their purpose. The fallout is of no importance to them whatsoever. It will require a public will to put an end to it. In sport, education and enforcement of the rules may have an impact on the demand side of the equation. The supply side needs concerted government action, not just here and there, but internationally, because the supply is international and the movement of the drugs involves many permeable borders. Governments have been less than effective, at the domestic level as well as in generating international consensus, and more importantly, action. Now is the time to do something about the problem. It is a problem.

12

Gene Doping

As if all the "regular" doping were not bad enough, we are about to see genetically modified athletes. I have no doubt that genetic manipulation experiments are already underway to improve sport performance. And it may become a reality sooner than we think possible!

Imagine the following scenario. It's August 2008, just weeks before the Olympics in Beijing. Eighteen-year-old Mike will be representing his country in the 400-meter race. A few months ago, he found a small, private gene-doping lab and underwent a procedure whereby synthetic genes were injected into his thigh muscles, altering his genetic makeup. Since then, his muscle mass has increased significantly, and he has knocked a full second off his personal best time. He's ready for the big race. He can't wait to beat the other athletes. They don't have his edge—at least, he doesn't think so. He believes his secret won't be detected by WADA, although he

CHAPTER TWELVE

can't be certain, and that worries him. But he doesn't worry too much about the risks of this yet-unproven technology. To Mike, winning is everything.

This sounds like science fiction, but, in reality, genetic engineering is right around the corner. In fact, some scientists have little doubt that gene-doped athletes, like Mike, will be competing in the 2008 Olympics in Beijing. Scary thought!

So, what exactly is gene doping? The original theory behind genetic engineering in medicine is to replace defective genes with healthy ones, with the hopes of some day treating or curing diseases such as cancer, cystic fibrosis and muscular dystrophy. But in sport, athletes will tinker with genes that increase strength or endurance. In gene doping, also called somatic cell modification, a doctor will intentionally inject synthetic genes into an athlete's cells through a carrier, such as a virus. This process modifies the cells and changes the athlete's genome—*forever*. Unlike drug doping, with gene doping, there's no going back. Once athletes are genetically modified, they are stuck with their new genes—*permanently*.

The implications of this new technology are mind-boggling. Imagine parents who want a sports champion juggling with the genetic makeup of their child at the embryonic stage. Imagine an arena full of athletes who all look the same. Imagine countries preselecting athletes at a very early age depending on their genetic makeup. Through genetic tracking, they may find that Tom may show a predisposition to sprinting, while Jane may be more of a marathon runner. Scientists can identify specific genes that may predict the innate athletic ability of an individual. But there are other factors to success. What if, after years of training, Tom and Jane don't turn out the way they are "supposed" to? How will this psychologically affect them?

Then there's the question of ethics and values. Will genetically modified athletes change the nature of sport? If winners are produced in science labs, what will happen to the human dimension of sport? What about the values, the fair play? What about the dreams of young athletes? With the constant pressure for athletic perfection, can this be the end of sport as we know it? The system will simply fall apart.

WADA CONFERENCE ON GENETIC DOPING

Maybe, just maybe, instead of playing catch-up with dopers, we can anticipate what may be coming and try to get there first with a reliable test.

While WADA is usually playing catch-up with drug dopers, it is in the unusual position of being if not one step ahead of the gene dopers, at least even with them. In March 2002, WADA organized a conference of leading genetic scientists to learn more about the work that was going on in the field of genetics. It was fascinating to learn that we may be on the threshold of discovering cures for diseases such as muscular dystrophy, diabetes and others. But, at the same conference, I also heard what I had long feared. One of the first inquiries that a team of genetic researchers had received came from a coach who wanted to know how he could use this technology on his athletes. He was talking about performance enhancement. It became quite apparent that some athletes, assisted by their coaches, were ready and anxious to gene-dope and would go to any length to do so. They simply didn't seem to care about the risks of this new and untested technology. Anything to win.

There were many questions raised at the conference. When genetic manipulation becomes a fact of life, where will this lead? This was far more serious than the use of anabolic steroids or EPO, the devils we know. How will society deal with the prospect of "breeding" basketball teams in the future? What ethical guidelines will be placed on research and implementation of genetic projects? How will they be enforced? What are the differences between genetic design, genetic modification, genetic treatment and genetic enhancement? Could sports leaders be helpful to the scientific community as policies are developed in this field?

There were some questions that only experts in this field could answer. They were in the forefront of the new science, so they had a better idea than did we, in the sport community, of what lies ahead. They knew the risks. They knew how drugs, such as EPO, which had been developed to treat illnesses, have also been used for performance enhancement. They knew what issues, ethical and otherwise, society as a whole must face. We had no idea where their science would take humanity nor how these advances might be perverted by those who would de-humanize sport. Medical miracles may become nightmares as gene doping enters the sports arena.

So, here we are, at the beginning of a possible brave new world. How close we are is a matter of speculation. Ted Friedmann, a leading authority on gene engineering and a member of WADA's Gene Doping Committee says that the National Institute of Health (NIH) Recombinant DNA Advisory Committee of the United States has not yet approved any gene transfer studies other than for the purpose of treating disease. But this is, despite its importance, only one agency in one country. The same kinds of scientists who developed THG may well be ready to develop this technology and apply it to sport for profit. They may be in the United States, or China, or somewhere else. But it is reasonable to assume that they will soon exist somewhere, and be willing to use the technology for performance enhancement. In fact, as I write this, they undoubtedly already do exist, and I would be willing to bet that some unscrupulous scientists have already attempted to use genetic modification technology—and, almost certainly, without the necessary study to determine the full risks of that use.

REGULATING GENE TRANSFER TECHNOLOGY

Don't wait to set up the regulatory framework. It must be done now.

The time to grab hold of the issue of gene transfer technology is now, through regulations and enforcement at the laboratory level, in the rules for clinical testing and in the application of proven technology. It is far easier to prevent a problem than it is to solve it. Or, as the old saw goes, an ounce of prevention is worth a pound of cure.

I hope that governments, regulatory agencies, academic institutions, professional governing bodies and the public at large will insist on regulating gene transfer technology, nationally and internationally. This application of science may come perilously close to how we define our humanity, so its implications deserve the most careful study. The misuse of therapeutic drugs is one thing; changing the genetic makeup of people is quite another. I also hope that sport will be given a seat at the policy-making table.

TESTING FOR GENE DOPING

The dilemma is, how do you test for something that may not yet exist and that may be indistinguishable from the real thing once it does?

CHAPTER TWELVE

I also hope that as the technology moves from the labs to clinical trials, the process will include developing tests to detect the use of gene doping technology. I am aware that a gene is a gene and that it may be impossible to detect the altered from the natural, but there may be (and probably are) indirect indicators that will provide sufficient scientific certainty to allow them to be used for testing purposes. After all, with many of the drugs we test for, it is the metabolites that we find rather than the actual drug itself.

At the conference in 2002, we had an initial fright when scientists stated that it would not be possible to test for genetic doping because it would be impossible to tell the difference between natural and "man-made" genes. Well, possibly, a muscle biopsy might show something, but even that might not be certain. And which muscle would you select to sample? It would be difficult to get athletes to agree to undergo this surgical procedure prior to a competition. It was concluded that muscle biopsies were probably too invasive to be applied in sport. This was devastating news.

I pressed on. I said the detection method could be indirect so long as the scientists were scientifically satisfied with the result. This started a whole buzz of conversation among them, and I left the conference with far more confidence that there would be a reliable test for gene doping before long. The human organism is so finely balanced that if you alter here, there will be an impact somewhere else. We just need to recognize what and where it is.

We kept in regular touch with the scientists as their work progressed. In the meantime, even though we still did not have detection capabilities, genetic doping and transfers were added to the List of the new World Anti-Doping Code, which was adopted in March 2003. This was not the first time that we had put something on the List even though there was no test. We wanted to give an early warning to potential gene dopers. The risk of this, of course, is that it might be taken as an invitation to use the technique because there is no test. The uncertainty revolves around how soon we will have a test. The Code contains a provision that allows us to go back eight years so that once a gene-doping test is perfected, we can re-test previous results. We also established a sub-committee to deal with genetic doping and agreed to fund research projects in the field.

GETTING CLOSER

The scientists seized the challenge and in a remarkably short period have made significant progress toward having a test that may be ready by the time the genetic dopers appear.

In December 2005, we held another symposium with the genetic community as a whole at the Karolinska Institute in Stockholm. The symposium was scheduled a week prior to the selection of the Nobel Prize. This evening was, for certain, the closest I would ever get to a Nobel Prize, but at the formal dinner, I expressed the thought that one or more of the scientists in the room might well get to a future Nobel banquet on their own merits. We have been fortunate indeed to have had the support of some extraordinary intellectual horsepower as we try to ensure that worthwhile therapeutic science is not misapplied to help cheating in sport.

As I mentioned, it would not be stretching the imagination too much to assume that some attempts have already been made to apply gene transfer technology to sport. The chemistry is not that complicated. It would not require a Ph.D. in order to manage the process, and any one of ten thousand laboratories could attempt it. Of course, attempting and succeeding are quite different. Many

CHAPTER TWELVE

things can go wrong, and the risks include death, which has occurred even under the most carefully supervised therapeutic medical conditions.

The symposium was generally positive about having tests in place by the time gene doping was available in sport. It is a huge advantage to be there as the science develops. A particularly encouraging outcome of the symposium was the call for the adoption of codes of professional conduct that would prevent gene doping in non-therapeutic circumstances.

On the dark side came news in early 2006, during a trial in Germany involving a coach, of e-mail correspondence, introduced as evidence, relating to a substance called Repoxygen that might be used for genetic manipulation. Repoxygen has the ability to stimulate the production of red blood cells in the same manner as EPO, but the difference is that it is inserted directly into the genetic makeup of the athlete. The coach had noted in his correspondence that Repoxygen was very difficult to come by, and it was not possible from the correspondence to know whether he was aware of any actual use. The British company that had developed Repoxygen had announced that it would not be producing or distributing it any further. I do not know whether there are other laboratories that can produce it. The worrying part is that there continue to be those who are willing to use any means, with whatever the risks, simply to get an advantage in sport.

At the time of our Stockholm symposium, an article on genetic enhancement in sport by a group of academics was ever-so-carefully coordinated to be released at the same time as the symposium was held. The thesis of the article was that genetic enhancement in sport was perfectly fine and, believe it or not, even fully justified. Anything for publicity. I just hope that such positions do not lead some athletes and scientists in that direction without an informed understanding of the inherent risks. Sometimes I wonder what color the sky is in the universes of certain scholars.

HUMANS, NOT MUTANTS

Science is science, and knowledge is knowledge. I do not mean to suggest that either should be limited. I believe in the advancement of knowledge in all fields. But we must be responsible for the ethical application of that knowledge. Understanding the power locked in the atom is an exciting scientific discovery. Using that knowledge to build nuclear power-generating plants can be seen as positive, but using it to create an atomic bomb is perhaps the ultimate negative use. Understanding the properties of certain germs is important and can save lives, but using that knowledge for biological warfare is terrifying.

The risks connected to the use of traditional drugs may seem minor compared with what might happen when you experiment with genetic manipulation. Who knows what the side effects may be of increasing muscle mass by fifteen percent with no need to exercise? Who knows what may happen if the myostatin mechanism that limits muscle size ceases to operate, muscle growth becomes unrestrained by natural processes and the results are like the German child of enormous proportion, or the Belgian beef experiment that produced bigger and denser beef cattle, far outside the normal parameters? Who knows what may happen if the trigger mechanisms that cause the muscle growth do not work, do not start or do not stop when expected?

I want to keep this in perspective. Gene transfer technology may be wonderful and desirable to treat illnesses, but it should not be used on perfectly healthy

CHAPTER TWELVE

athletes merely to cheat by enhancing their performance. Society is built on an ethical platform, as is sport. Those platforms should be sturdy enough, sufficiently defined and sufficiently enforced to deal with advances in the sciences.

I want gold medals to be presented to athletes who earned them honestly, not to their secret pharmacists or gene transfer technologists.

I want sport, not a circus.

I want athletes, not gladiators.

I want human beings, not mutants.

Don't you?

13 See No Evil, Hear No Evil, Speak No Evil

Too many people know what is going on, but they seem to be paralyzed and unable to speak out. The athletes know who is doping; the coaches know who is doping; many of the media know who is doping. Why do they not say something?

Part of the problem with doping cases in many sports is that the people in charge often would rather not know the truth. To them, each positive test reflects badly on them and on the sport itself. So, they are quite happy to keep the bad news from being delivered in the first place and, if delivered, to keep it under wraps as much as possible. There is precious little effort to use positive tests as evidence to detect cheaters and take cheaters out of competition so that clean athletes have a better chance to achieve the results they deserve. As long as sport organizations are not willing to assume the responsibility of cleaning up sports, the blot of doping will be that much harder to remove.

CHAPTER THIRTEEN

L'AFFAIRE LANCE

When the allegations of Lance Armstrong's use of EPO became public, both Armstrong and the International Cycling Union (UCI) had the same reaction: how did this embarrassing information find its way into the press? But no one seemed interested in finding out whether the allegations were true or not.

The recent revelations regarding Lance Armstrong are a case in point. On August 23, 2005, the French daily newspaper *L'Equipe* published an explosive feature headlined "Le mensonge Armstrong" ("The Armstrong Lie"). The article claimed to have matched doping control forms signed by Armstrong during the 1999 Tour de France with positive EPO results. Armstrong was no ordinary rider. Earlier, he had won his seventh consecutive Tour de France, something no one in history had ever accomplished. He was the King of the Tour. Was he now to be disgraced and exposed as a cheater? Would the Tour authorities try to recover any prize money? Had the string of successes all been an act, a charade, on the part of an accomplished liar? It was a stunning revelation. But was it true, or merely some scandalous media invention?

I had been aware of what turned out to be part of the story because the French laboratory had advised WADA that it still had some frozen urine samples on hand from the 1998 and 1999 Tours. The lab, one of the leading laboratories in the world in the field of EPO research and testing, had been improving their test for EPO and wanted to try it out on the older samples. WADA was interested, as it was useful for us to have an idea of when and where EPO was being used in sport, even if that usage had occurred prior to the establishment of WADA at the end of 1999. We were also curious to know whether the International Cycling Union (UCI) had used the Festina scandal in 1998 to make its testing regime for EPO more effective, even though the test had then not yet been perfected. The comparison between the two years would be valuable. One of WADA's mandates is to identify doping in sport, not to protect the identities of athletes who dope, so we advised the lab that we would be interested in the analysis. In due course, we received the results. There were a number of the samples that showed the usage of EPO, but since we received only the code numbers of the samples, we did not know the identities of the athletes involved. Nevertheless, we thought the results might be part of a larger puzzle. At the very least, we thought that the UCI would be interested in knowing which of its athletes had been using the prohibited EPO, since the UCI had the code numbers and the names of the athletes assigned these codes.

Publication of the story brought immediate reaction from Armstrong and the UCI, but the focus of the reaction was how this embarrassing information had found its way into the press. No one seemed the slightest bit interested in discussing whether the allegations of Armstrong's (and others) drug use were true or not. Fingers were pointed everywhere. The UCI all but accused the newspaper of having stolen the documents. The French laboratory and French government were accused of leaks, ethical breaches and anti-Americanism. WADA was accused of being the source of the leaks, since it had received a copy of the test results. But none of the finger-pointing was directed at either Armstrong or the UCI. Since the newspaper had published copies of the doping control forms, it seemed natural to wonder who had provided them. WADA did not have copies of these, but who did? The original copy of each form was retained by the UCI, and the athlete, the French cycling federation and the French ministry each kept a copy.

CHAPTER THIRTEEN

The laboratory received a copy, with no identification of the athlete, only a code number. If a test is positive, the code is then matched by the cycling authorities with the doping control form, and the disciplinary process begins. Each copy of the doping control form is numbered so that one can identify whose copy it is. The French ministry had destroyed its copies of the 1999 forms several years earlier, as, I believe, had the French cycling federation. Armstrong had certainly not given his copies of the forms to the press. This left the UCI as the only possible source.

I was at my desk in my law office a few days after the story broke, when Lance Armstrong and his agent, Bill Stapleton, called. He knew I had seen the *L'Equipe* article since I had been interviewed by the media about this issue and commented in general terms only because I did not have all the facts. I told Armstrong that I thought he had a problem that was more than the usual "he said/she said" variety of doping allegations that surrounded him. I said that there might well be a case for him to answer. But, like everyone else, Armstrong was only interested in identifying the source of the information, not the substance of it. They had three or four questions to ask, such as what contact WADA had had with the laboratory and whether WADA had funded the research. I said I would try to get answers for them, which I did and which I e-mailed to Armstrong.

Now, I do not know for sure whether Armstrong was guilty or not of using EPO during the 1999 Tour de France, or thereafter, for that matter. I am romantic enough about sport that I long for genuine heroes, and nothing would make me happier than for the Armstrong legend to be true. Fine athlete, stricken by cancer, recovers and goes on to win one of the great cycling events, the Tour de France, not just once (an extraordinary feat in its own right) but a mind-boggling seven consecutive times. This should be a story for the ages. You could write off some of the rumors regarding his drug use to jealousy on the part of some disaffected individuals. You could say that his association with Dr. Michele Ferrari, the Italian doctor charged with doping fraud in sport, was unfortunate, but it did not necessarily mean that Armstrong himself was shopping for the same services as those for which the doctor was charged.

I have never met Armstrong. The first indirect contact we had occurred a couple of years earlier when I saw an open letter from him in the media complaining about some remarks I had made about the drug problem in cycling. I think I had said in an interview that everyone knew there were riders in the Tour de France who were doping, which when translated into French appeared as "les" riders, which Armstrong misunderstood as me having said "all the riders" were using drugs. I expect I answered in the same open-letter format but cannot remember what I said. A year or so later, my phone rang, and the person on the other end of the line said, "Dick, this is Lance Armstrong." He talked about his love for his sport. I told him that I thought his sport had a serious drug problem and that sometimes you had to be willing to apply tough love in situations that called for it. The call was inconclusive, and we left it with vague assurances that we would stay in touch. I doubt that the call was without some purpose on Armstrong's part, but what it was intended to accomplish, I do not know. That was the last I heard from Armstrong until after the Tour de France revelations surfaced in August 2005.

But something that cannot be ignored is the reaction of both the Armstrong camp and the UCI to the published story, which combines allegations with what appear to be copies of authentic documents. These facts are either true or they are false; there is no middle ground. If they are false, it should be easy to demonstrate that and, once and for all, dispel the suspicions that swirl around Armstrong. Maybe the documents are, for example, not copies of the originals, or maybe they have been altered. The original documents are in the possession of the UCI, and perhaps even Armstrong has kept his copies. After all, they are critically important documents in a sport that has a known doping problem and for an individual who was tested at least fifteen times during the 1999 Tour. Or maybe he could say that the urine that was tested was not his, although he might then have to suggest how someone had exchanged someone else's urine for his. Or perhaps he could challenge the technical analysis performed by the French laboratory by demonstrating that it was improperly done. The French laboratory still has enough of the urine samples to do further analysis to determine whether the appropriate scientific standards have been applied. As a clincher, Armstrong could offer to provide a DNA sample that could be compared with the DNA in the samples that were analyzed by the laboratory to show that the urine could not possibly have been provided by him. He has said that he "knows" it was not his urine, so it ought to be a slam dunk. You would think that Armstrong himself would love to put an end to all the rumors that surround him in order to demonstrate that he was not cheating when he won the Tour de France. The UCI should also jump at such a chance to show that the innuendo surrounding its star is nothing more than a tissue of lies. I suggested exactly that to Armstrong soon after the *L'Equipe* article appeared, saying I was sure that would be better than spending money on lawyers. Instead, I got a letter from Armstrong's lawyer, saying that I was violating his client's rights!

LANCE ON *LARRY KING LIVE*

Many Americans feel that the French resent the fact that the Tour de France was not won by a French rider, but

> *instead by an American. This one-dimensional theory conveniently overlooks the fact that there has not been a French winner of the event in some twenty years, as well as the fact that another American rider, Greg LeMond, was a triple winner of the event (1986, 1989, 1990). There is no convincing evidence that Armstrong is disliked in France just because he is an American.*

My sense is that Armstrong is withdrawing from most fields of play, except in the United States where he is still uncritically admired. There, the home crowd is ready to buy the story that the 1999 Tour de France revelations were an anti-American ploy on the part of the French and, if you believe what Armstrong says, a witch-hunt on my part directed at him. He made a rather unconvincing early appearance, August 25, 2005, on *Larry King Live*. Unfortunately, only Bob Costas had a few hard-hitting questions.

> **Armstrong:**
> OK, you know a guy in a French-Parisian laboratory opens up your sample, you know, Jean-Francis so-and-so, and he tests it. Nobody's there to observe. No protocol was followed. And then you get a call from a newspaper that says we found you to be positive six times for EPO. Well, since when did newspapers start governing sports?
>
> **Bob Costas:**
> Here's the head of the World Anti-Doping Agency, Richard Pound, a long-time Olympic official. He said this week, "It's not a he said/she said scenario. There were documents. Unless the documents are forgeries or manipulations, it's a case that has to be answered."

CHAPTER THIRTEEN

Armstrong:
You know what? It is absolutely a case of he said/she said. What else can it be? Do you think I'm going to trust some guy in a French lab to open my samples and say they're positive and announce that to the world and not give me the chance to defend myself? That's ludicrous. There is no way you can do that.

Armstrong continued to cast doubt on the effectiveness of the tests, the storage of the samples, the stability of the stored samples and the lack of scientific data, about which he had no information whatsoever. He admitted that cycling perhaps does have a "culture" of doping and a long history of doping and that some efforts were made after the Festina scandal in 1998. He said that there were still samples from twenty, twenty-five, thirty years ago, but that they (the French) just happened to pick 1999. I doubt this is true, but even if true, it was beside the point. He then referred to a rule in the WADA Code that states that when there is only one sample left, it must remain anonymous and could never be made public. It could be used only for experimentation, only if the athlete gives approval and, in that case, it would have to be anonymous forever. Someone, along the way, he said, had violated two very serious WADA codes. In fact, no one had. Armstrong conveniently forgot to mention that WADA had not even been created in 1999 when he provided the samples. He disputed that the French laboratory still had the samples. On the other hand, if it is conceded that WADA has some role to play, then maybe all of the rules should apply, even the right to go back eight years to retest samples, including 1999.

Next, Armstrong appeared on *Saturday Night Live*, where partisan mocking of the French continued. The theory for U.S. consumption seems to be that everything behind the revelations is a reflection of the view that the French resent the fact that the Tour de France was not won by a French rider but instead by an American. This one-dimensional characterization conveniently overlooks the fact that there has not been a French winner of the event in some twenty years, as well as the fact that another American rider, Greg LeMond, was a triple winner of the event (1986, 1989, 1990). Politically, the United States and France have disagreed over the Iraq war and other things, but there is no convincing evidence that Armstrong is disliked in France just because he is an American.

UCI "INVESTIGATES"

> *The UCI presented many difficulties for WADA. Our original desire was for the UCI, as the international federation responsible for cycling, to take charge of the matter and to investigate all the facts, determine whether there had been doping and act accordingly. But the UCI was totally preoccupied with* how the information became public, not with the *who, what, where, when* and *why of the actual doping.*

After the revelations in *L'Equipe*, the UCI agreed to conduct an investigation. It appointed a Dutch lawyer, Emile Vrijman, to conduct an "independent" investigation of the matter. But when we asked him to advise us as to the terms of reference of his examination, he did not reply to us. The ability to gain full and unrestricted access to all of the relevant documents would depend on whether Armstrong took any legal action to sue *L'Equipe* for libel. Only then would the documents have become available. But the drop-dead date for that action was November 23, 2005, and it came and went with no action by Armstrong.

CHAPTER THIRTEEN

He has never been shy about resorting to lawsuits, but most have been settled out of court and, generally, no terms of settlement are disclosed.

The UCI position has presented many difficulties for WADA. Our original desire was for the UCI, as the international federation responsible for cycling, to take charge of the matter, investigate all the facts, determine whether there had been doping and act accordingly. We understand that it may be too late to do much about the past, but the UCI ought to be aware of any doping and, if a test is found to be positive, to put at least a mental or informal marker against the result, somewhat the way the IOC, along with the rest of the world, has done regarding some of the former East German results and MLB should do with some of its records.

The then president of UCI, Hein Verbruggen, admitted that one of the six dope test forms came from the UCI. However, he maintained that the other five published Armstrong forms that were also linked to positive EPO results must have come from some other source. Verbruggen went so far as to publicly suggest a number of possibilities (excluding the possibility that the forms might have come from the UCI itself), pointing fingers at WADA, the French laboratory (nonsense, since the laboratory does not get copies of the documents that identify the riders), the French ministry of sport (which destroyed its copies of the forms several years ago) or a WADA employee.

Several weeks after the publication of the story, I obtained copies of the forms for fifteen tests performed on Armstrong during the 1999 Tour de France. Each of these forms is the copy belonging to the UCI and could only have come from the UCI and with its express consent. No one suggested that there had been a burglary at UCI headquarters. I showed these copies of the forms to Verbruggen and IOC president Jacques Rogge during the

Turin Olympics. I also said, between colleagues, that I was willing to accept Verbruggen's assurances that he had not personally given the forms to the reporter. I do not know whether he had believed that the other forms had, in fact, come from the UCI, but with the copies I showed him, it was impossible to argue that there could have been any other possible explanation or source.

The UCI then commenced an internal investigation, which concluded that a member of its medical team had, indeed, given all the forms to the reporter. The employee was suspended and Verbruggen told me he would certainly be fired as a consequence of giving the forms. A statement was issued by the UCI on February 27, acknowledging that it was the source of all the documents referred to in *L'Equipe*, despite its earlier public statements to the contrary. Nor was the employee fired—a month later, he was reinstated.

Vrijman issued his formal report on May 31, 2006. It was, as we had suspected from the outset, shockingly incomplete and unreliable. WADA has issued a statement identifying the many mis-statements of fact, insinuations, errors and unreasoned conclusions. According to the report, none of the fault is attributed to the UCI, but is laid at the doorstep of WADA (and me personally) and the French laboratory. In Turin during the Games, Verbruggen told me that Vrijman's report would be very critical of WADA and me, and that it would destroy our credibility in the fight against doping in sport. I said, with a raised eyebrow, I was surprised to learn that this conclusion had been reached, because Vrijman, his countryman, had never contacted WADA for any information and had not even answered our inquiry of several months ago regarding his mandate. By sheer coincidence, shortly after I returned from Turin, some questions arrived from Vrijman, which we answered. There were no follow-up questions.

CHAPTER THIRTEEN

During a visit to UCI headquarters in Switzerland on April 13, 2006, the UCI president advised me that the Vrijman report had arrived the previous day, but that it was quite thick and he had not yet read it. No one has yet commented on the remarkable fact that the UCI apparently had the "independent" report in its possession for six weeks before it was publicly issued, nor on whether there were discussions between the UCI and Vrijman as to its contents. This casts serious doubts as to the independent nature of the report and raises questions as to the possible role the UCI had in the report reaching the conclusions it contains.

So, where are we? The UCI has been totally preoccupied with how the information became public. We now know how the information got out, but there are still the facts to be dealt with. Were the samples Armstrong's or not? Did they disclose the presence of EPO or not? All the concerted attention to the manner of disclosure cannot obliterate the need for an answer to these questions. Was Armstrong cheating during the 1999 Tour de France? Who were the other riders who tested positive in the same event? The UCI knows the identities of these riders, unless it no longer has the other forms, but it would be odd indeed if the only forms it had kept from 1999 had been Armstrong's.

It is beyond my comprehension how the UCI thought that a report of this nature would do anything to clarify the situation. None of the anti-doping experts who have commented on the scientific portion of the report has any confidence in the credentials of the Dutch expert retained by Vrijman to declare that the French laboratory had improperly performed the tests, that the tests were unreliable and that there had been other mistakes in the analysis. I think it will become even clearer over time that there was indeed EPO in those samples in which the laboratory concluded there was and that the independent scientific conclusions of the expert used by Vrijman are, plain and simple, wrong.

See No Evil, Hear No Evil, Speak No Evil

The effort to clear Armstrong and the other athletes of the charges will lead to even more pressing questions. The unwillingness of the UCI to acknowledge its responsibilities to act on the available information will do nothing to add to its own credibility, which has recently taken another massive hit in the disclosure of widespread doping in Spain that has disrupted the 2006 Tour de France, involving not just the riders at the back of the peloton, but the presumptive successors to Armstrong. As for WADA, we simply want to know whether there was drug use in the 1999 Tour de France. The biased nature of the Vrijman report has heightened, rather than relieved, our concerns. And, in my view, Armstrong should have known better than to trumpet that he had been exonerated by a report that was so badly flawed and clearly not independent. Its independence was dismissed out of hand by the IOC president, Jacques Rogge, when Armstrong tried to use the report as a basis to have me removed as the head of WADA. This kind of behavior does nothing to help his credibility. It makes me think of the line from *Hamlet*: "The [laddy] doth protest too much, methinks."

I do not want to suggest that cycling is the only federation with drug problems, nor that it is by any means the least committed to stopping drug use in its sport. I have used it as an example, since the Armstrong affair has attracted more than its share of media attention. It has led to a considerable amount of public and private confrontation with the UCI and other cycling organizations, combined with threats of lawsuits and unspecified disciplinary proceedings directed at WADA and me personally for having drawn forceful attention to the situation. These have been unfortunate reactions. One would think that the solution would have been to try to work together with WADA, taking advantage of the combination of sport and governments, in a joint effort to improve the situation.

CHAPTER THIRTEEN

Even the most committed supporters of cycling admit, perhaps only privately, that there is a problem of doping in cycling and that the efforts of cycling officials to clean up the sport, including testing, have not been successful. At my meeting with the UCI in April 2006, I almost fell off my chair when Hein Verbruggen said that the UCI had so few positive drug tests that they had concluded there was not a drug problem in cycling after all and they were giving serious thought to reducing the number of tests they performed. In the latter part of 2005, an Ipsos survey was released in Europe, showing that almost eighty percent of respondents considered cycling as the sport with which doping is most associated. The main countries surveyed were the big cycling countries—France, Germany, Italy and Spain. This is a remarkable consensus, especially on a continent that has shown a fairly *laissez-faire* attitude to drug use in one of its favorite sports. It has always been known that drug use has been a feature of cycling and the Tour de France, but this was driven home during the 1998 Tour when the French police arrested members of the Festina team for doping offenses. An even more spectacular and wide-ranging drug scandal uncovered by the Spanish authorities in 2006 may provide yet another opportunity for cycling to finally acknowledge the existence of a serious problem and develop more effective anti-doping programs.

The new UCI president, Pat McQuaid, refers to the problem as the "scourge" of doping in his sport. I agree and simply add that the same scourge exists elsewhere and that everyone needs to work together to make progress in stamping it out. Doping in sport is a real problem and it will not be solved by ignoring it. Or by shooting the messenger.

See No Evil, Hear No Evil, Speak No Evil

WHERE ARE THE ATHLETES?

> *We need more athletes to speak out about doping. They are on the inside and know who is doing what. There is no reason why they should meekly accept systematic cheating from fellow competitors. I have no compunction whatsoever in taking whatever advantage we can of any knowledge, however we acquire it, from those on the inside.*

There is another group that knows what is going on in sport—the athletes. They cannot help but be aware of drug use by their fellow competitors. Athletes who play fair know they are being cheated by others, but as a group they are strangely silent about what they know. They refuse to talk about this issue. The doping athletes won't admit that they use dope, and those who do not dope don't want to talk about what the cheaters are doing. What happens in the locker room stays in the locker room. They have seen other athletes shunned and ridiculed as whiners when they speak out against what may be going on. They do not want to become shuttlecocks in some media exercise. And they don't want to be sued by aggressive cheaters in case they can't prove what they know to the satisfaction of a court or jury. They just keep their heads down and get on with life, however imperfect and unfair it may be. I understand that they cannot expect sports officials to disqualify competitors simply on their say-so, but there are many ways to draw attention to the problems and to help point the way to those in a position to do something about it.

On the eve of the 2002 Olympic Winter Games in Salt Lake City, there was a much-publicized apparent dispute between me and Canadian cross-country skier Beckie Scott. Scott has long been an outspoken critic of doping in her

CHAPTER THIRTEEN

sport. She sometimes even gave the impression that she thought that sports officials and WADA were not doing enough about the problem. My response to this was that without some credible evidence of doping, we could not disqualify an athlete based only on suspicion or unsupported accusations. This was immediately perceived to be a fight between Scott and me, which it clearly was not.

Scott had every right to be outraged at the level of cheating going on in her sport and to call attention to it. However, she was not right to suggest that the authorities were not doing enough to combat the practice. The cross-country-skiing authorities had come rather late to the party, but, in their defense, it was only in 2000 that a viable test for EPO had been devised, and they had acted quickly in 2001 at the world championships.

It was not at all fair to say that WADA and sports officials were less than active in this fight. After all, had it not been for the "old guys in the suits," Scott would not have eventually received the silver and gold medals that were originally presented to her doping competitors in the 2002 Olymics. This was achieved as a direct result of those committed to the fight against doping in sport. Scott has since joined the WADA Athlete Committee and will be able to continue that same fight alongside us. We are delighted to have someone with such a profile at the table. During the 2006 Games, in addition to her splendid results in the competitions, she was elected by the Olympic athletes participating in Turin as a member of the IOC Athletes' Commission. In that capacity, she has also been elected as a full member of the IOC.

I hope this will encourage other athletes to speak out. There is no reason why they should meekly accept systematic cheating from their fellow competitors. They may get an encouraging leg up from the impact that Kelli White has had in being willing (albeit as part of the sanction for her participation in the Balco scheme) to say what she knows about drug use in her sport. It was her testimony that led to the conviction of Tim Montgomery and Chrystie Gaines for the use of THG. At WADA, we encourage anyone with knowledge to come forward so that we will have a better idea of where to look and what to look for when we do our testing. As it pertains to athletes in particular, I do not necessarily expect them to make specific allegations or to come out with public declarations regarding athletes they suspect of doping. They may be unwilling to speak "on the record" for fear of being sued, especially where there are financial interests at stake. But they can certainly lead the way to more targeted testing if, for example, they know what athletes in certain sports or countries are doing, how they do it and when, and that will have the same impact. I have no compunction whatsoever in taking whatever advantage we can of any knowledge, however we acquire it, from those on the inside.

COACHES' CORNER

Whenever there is widespread doping in sport, the coaches must be aware of it. If they are not, they simply are not doing their jobs.

Athletes may or may not know what is going on with drug use in sport, but the coaches definitely know. Instead of monkey see, monkey do, they should, through their associations or individually, be pointing out what is going on, drawing attention to it and acting to ensure that the responsible authorities are active in combating it. For years, it was clear

CHAPTER THIRTEEN

that there had been systematic doping in East Germany and east bloc countries and that such activities had been copied at a private level in the western democracies. Perhaps that had led to a stalemate, since everyone was guilty of something. But the stalemate had been the result of being unwilling to confront the problem openly. Instead, the coaches, too, went underground to match what their professional counterparts were doing, or they just gritted their teeth and watched their equally talented athletes getting whipped by artificially enhanced competitors. It would be interesting to know why there was no concerted outcry in the rest of the world until the Chinese athletes suddenly began to perform at levels they had not previously reached, especially in swimming, where the presence of former East German coaches was not a coincidence. Be that as it may, there was no doubt that the coaching fraternity knew who among them used doping to improve their athletes' performances. The same is true today.

It is refreshing to see that the German authorities have decided to prosecute some of the coaches who had been involved in the former regime with the systematic doping of athletes, particularly those who were minors. Although convictions usually result in only minor fines, these do have a symbolic impact. Also, they may show the way for other countries to do something along the same lines. But, I suspect that cynical political considerations will probably incline them to leave the sleeping dogs at rest, rather than embarrass the national conscience. The Italians have had to deal with entire soccer teams that have been doped, but they seem strangely unable to come to grips with a solution, nor, frankly, to have much appetite to find one. Revelations of similar team-wide doping in American professional football have led nowhere, although the doctor involved with the Carolina Panthers recently had his medical license revoked and was convicted for doping offences. It is not credible that the coaches of these teams were unaware of what was going on with their athletes—not credible at all.

HYPOCRITES OF THE HIPPOCRATIC OATH

> *I think we should publish a list of those TUEs that are rejected, revealing the names of the athletes, the names of the physicians who issued them and why we rejected them. Why shouldn't the doctors be exposed as the cheating assistants they are?*

There is, in the end, not much good that can be said of medical practitioners who are complicit in doping. In fact, there should be little but contempt for them. To assist with such activities when they know the purpose is cheating not therapeutic, and can, in fact, be dangerous to the patient's health, goes against their Hippocratic oath. Such conduct can be something as simple as granting a TUE for the use of a prohibited substance when there is no genuine medical need for it. I have often commented in public about the astonishing percentage of brave and dedicated athletes in international sport who seem to have arrived at the pinnacle of performance despite a medically acknowledged condition of asthma! This requires them to take beta-2 agonists to help them breathe, all cheerfully prescribed by physicians. Prescribing insulin for the wrong purpose falls into the same category. Issuing questionable TUEs has become so commonplace that we have had to establish an international TUE committee to review all TUEs in order to determine which are justified and which are not. I think we should publish a list of those that are rejected, revealing the names of the athletes, the names of the physicians who issued them and why we rejected them. Why shouldn't these physicians be exposed as the agents of cheating they are?

CHAPTER THIRTEEN

The lamest excuse that we hear from physicians regarding drug use is that it is better for the athletes to be using the prohibited substances under the care of a doctor than to be using them on their own account, unsupervised. The ethical barrier here is so permeable that it barely exists. Everything is wrapped in the rationalization that their only concern is the health of the athlete and minimization of the risks to them of using the drugs. They say that the athletes may use them anyway, which is not their business, and that they simply are monitoring their physical condition. This noble sentiment overlooks the fact that there were doctors in East Germany and almost certainly elsewhere that supervised the administration of drugs in industrial quantities to athletes where they neither knew nor apparently cared what the side effects might be. The bottom line is that it is unprofessional to act in such a manner. Professional bodies should, as a matter of ethical principle, discipline practitioners who act in such a manner. I hope this will be one of the eventual positive results that will come from the recently adopted UNESCO International Convention on Doping in Sport. Governments have the power to regulate in this area, while sport organizations cannot.

THE PUBLIC: WAKENING THE SLEEPING GIANT

Like it or not, sports stars are heroes and idols to our kids. Our kids copy their heroes' behavior. That's why we have to encourage the stars to be good role models, both on and off the field.

Nothing can resist the tide of an idea whose time has come. I cannot say for certain that the public has yet fully embraced the idea of drug-free sport, but there are signs that an awakening is underway. There is an increased awareness that there is, in fact, a problem and that it has not been sufficiently dealt with by those responsible for it. Almost no one would condone athletes doing and taking whatever they want while training and participating in sport. Imagine someone standing up to say, "We do not care what our athletes do and what they take to get ready. Whatever level of drugs and violence appeals to them is fine with us, and we hope to set a fine example for the youth of the world." This would be completely unacceptable. On the other hand, we have shown a remarkable willingness to accept that the conduct in real life is not too removed from the extreme example I have just suggested. There are often obsessions about breaking records, in which the excitement of the competition is nothing and the record everything. I don't know about you, but when I watch a 100 meter race, I watch the race and then look to see what the time was. I do not watch the clock to see when it stops and then try to figure out who may have won.

Many of the professional sports have become entertainment first and sport second. They are businesses that feed on whatever interests the public from time to time. If the public wants bigger, stronger and faster athletes and more and more violence in their entertainment, that is what they get. How this is delivered is less important than the fact that the businesses are willing to provide it. What the gladiator class does to prepare for the few hours of diversion for the masses does not seem to matter, and no one cares what the price is for those who provide the entertainment. The average career in the NFL is four years, and a huge percentage of those who fall within that average lose their jobs due to injuries. When you see the size and speed of the athletes, it is small wonder. Human joints are not designed for the stress and impact today's players suffer. A few seconds of applause may be the only eulogy for a player who will leave the field on a stretcher, never to return.

CHAPTER THIRTEEN

At one level, we all know this, but on another, we are not much better than the Roman crowds diverted by the carnage in a coliseum. I have often wondered whether television has had the effect of turning everything about life into a video game, where what happens is not real. I do not mean "not real" in the sense that what we see never happens, but that it has no close connection with our normal lives. Football players are players, to be sure, but we do not see them as people like us. They are characters playing a part that has been scripted for our amusement. I am sure that part of the reason is that you cannot see the players clearly. They all wear helmets and bulky armor-like equipment, which depersonalizes them, makes them less human, extends the gap between the humanity of the actors and the roles they play. This is the bad side of Vince Lombardi's famous quotation about winning being the only thing.

Hemmed in by society at large, we seem to crave violence, even vicarious violence, where "our" team is more violent than "your" team. We buy shirts and jackets to identify with the more spectacular characters. The first time this view of television struck me was when the first Gulf war was televised in 1991. It was the ultimate video game, where rockets, missiles and directed fire could be seen, but it seemed unreal. We were not able to see what was actually happening on the ground to real people—body parts and blood splattered among ruined buildings. This war seemed so unreal, and it ended so quickly—just like a game—that it was conceivable that the same video game could be played again and again, years later, with the same lack of involvement, in another country.

Perhaps I extrapolate too far. Perhaps not. But look around at the evolution of the sports we watch. Isn't there an increasing tendency to demand more powerful athletes, more violence? For that matter, look at the television programs in general and tell me that the public taste for violence is not increasing. Commercial television broadcasters want to please their viewing audiences. They depend on audiences for their ratings, and their ratings determine what they can charge for ads. If nobody watches, advertisers will spend their money elsewhere. Today, television has more choices than ever before. What you see is what people want.

How can you make a change?Vote with your TV's channel changer. Write to the advertising sponsor. Don't watch the "extreme" sports. Challenge the organizations that encourage such sports and permit their athletes to be violent. Challenge the professional leagues that say they have rules prohibiting the use of performance-enhancing drugs but take no real steps to enforce these rules. They treat their athletes with contempt, they treat you with contempt and they treat their games with contempt. In the long run, they will destroy their sports and erase the public trust in the integrity of sport.

14 Is There a Cure? My Ten-Step Program

Doping in sport can be beaten. We just need to persevere. But like that old sixties slogan states, "If you are not part of the solution, you are part of the problem."

Anyone who thinks there is no doping problem in sport is irrevocably divorced from reality. The problem is real, it does exist and it is more serious than most people care to believe. But there is a cure. It is not an easy one, but it is possible. Anyone who thinks the cure to doping in sport lies in an eight-second sound bite, though, is dreaming in color. Like any major problem, there are many facets. Defining it is certainly one of them. Figuring out what is and what is not doping and whether or not particular substances or methods ought to be prohibited is an important starting point. Another is how to get at the problem. And another is who should be part of the solution, which brings me back to the old slogan, sound bite though it appears, "If you are not part of the solution, you are part of the problem."

CHAPTER FOURTEEN

Dope is addicting, and so is doping. So, drawing on other addiction programs (such as Alcoholics Anonymous), I have come up with a ten-step program to get athletes, coaches, leagues, associations and so on off dope. It also helps "enablers" stop turning a blind eye.

STEP 1: END DENIAL AND RATIONALIZATION—THERE *IS* A PROBLEM

The first step in defining the cure for doping in sport is to acknowledge that there is a problem. Denial is one of the common features of addiction. Until you admit that there is a problem, it is not possible to cure it. In some cases, this denial is institutional. In others, it is by the people surrounding the athletes on whom the doping is practiced. The full range of psychological defenses is easily identified. The most common, after denial, is rationalization. "Everybody is doing it, so why shouldn't I?" Coaches say that their colleagues are doing it with their own athletes, so, to level the playing field, they have no alternative but to follow suit. The doctors who perform the procedures, administer the drugs or prescribe them soothe their consciences by saying that it is better for the athletes to do so under medical supervision to minimize the health risks. Officials look the other way, saying there are no means to control the situation.

I could have included a list of examples of doping over, say, the past ten years, but it would have doubled the size of the book. Trust me, there is a problem. It is not going to disappear by itself. It is too deeply ingrained in sport today. But, as is the case with all problems, there is a solution to the doping problem. It simply requires insight and commitment to implement the steps outlined here. There is no excuse for not trying.

STEP 2: IDENTIFY THE PROBLEM AND HOW BIG IT IS

What then, is the problem of doping in sport? The problem is actually fairly easy to define: There are people who do not care what sport is supposed to mean and who do not give a damn about the rules. Sport consists of competitive performances of certain activities according to a specified set of criteria. One of these rules is that certain drugs and methods for enhancing one's natural abilities are not permitted. Like other rules, there may be some degree of arbitrariness involved, although, if you look carefully enough, there is usually some degree of concern for the health of athletes implicit in every anti-doping rule. The health concerns may vary from substance to substance or from procedure to procedure, and some may be less risky than others, but, in the final analysis, that does not matter. If some substances or procedures are on the List that need not be there, there are ways of changing the List once there is a scientific consensus. In the long run, I think it is better to err on the side of caution than in the other direction. There are enough inherent risks in sport and competition already without adding drug risks to the equation, let alone throwing the dice with genetic manipulation.

The solution is that we agree not to use certain drugs and procedures. But some participants are sneaky and underhanded. They promise to follow the rules and pretend to do so, when they have no intention of doing so. They have every intention of trying to take advantage of other competitors by using drugs or methods that will enhance their performance beyond what it would otherwise be. No one does this to level a playing field. On the contrary, they want the field to be tilted their way. Everyone tries to aim for advantage, but there is no place in sport for those who try for

CHAPTER FOURTEEN

unfair advantage. There must be means of identifying the cheaters and getting rid of them. Identifying the problem is as simple as that.

STEP 3: LEARN WHY ATHLETES DOPE

There has not been enough research done to identify the reasons why athletes are willing to cheat and risk their health. It seems to me that understanding this is fundamental to designing the cure for doping. I admit that this is not that easy to research, especially since the very ones who could provide the best insights are those who are actually doping. Most are sufficiently paranoid about being exposed that they would either be unwilling to participate in a study or, if they did (perhaps to show they had nothing to hide), they would be unwilling to answer honestly. This is the conundrum for researchers: those they most want to understand are those who have the least interest in being truthful. The same is true of coaches, support staff and even the sports associations. If your future is at stake, you will be the most righteous of all in the public's eye.

Despite these reservations, WADA has recently funded some social research projects designed to try to get a more reliable handle on the underlying factors that go into the decision to dope. These pilot studies may provide some useful data that we can use in future studies. There are several likely factors that lead athletes to dope, but money is always cited as the principal reason. It is probably a dominating element, but only in those sports that have large enough monetary rewards to motivate athletes to cheat and endanger their health in order to win the money. This can happen among athletes making millions of dollars who begin to see the ends of their careers approaching and try to prolong their income stream as long as they can. But not all sports produce major income, even for the stars. One can make a good living from sport, but apart from a few stars in the major leagues or a handful of other sports, it is a good but not enormously pocketbook-enriching career. I often illustrate this by asking whether anyone has met a rich weightlifter. While recognizing the oversimplification, I use the example to show that there must be some other explanation for the willingness to risk their health, career and reputation that goes beyond mere money.

It goes beyond mere cash. There is a certain status that a winning athlete achieves through recognition, however narrow the base. There is no doubt that there seems to be inordinate respect for athletic prowess. Perhaps this comes from the ancient hunter-killer era of humankind, when homage was paid to the strongest in the group. Social status and advantages, such as apartments, cars and other benefits were known to be linked to sport success in the former east bloc countries. The stakes may have been high enough to allow the athletes to rationalize their use of drugs.

Is there some general kind of neurosis that attacks all athletes who live in the crucible of competition, where the tiniest differences mean the difference between the fame attaching to a winner and the relative obscurity of being anything but the winner? At the 2006 Winter Olympics in Turin, in one of the women's speed skating events, the first three places were separated by a total of six one-hundredths of a second. The differences are so minute that if athletes think there may be something "out there" that can give them the tiny extra boost that may tip the scales in their direction, they may be willing to take any risk to get the edge that they think will make the difference between winning and not winning. In the course of this search, the rules may be forgotten or ignored.

CHAPTER FOURTEEN

Coaches and officials are likely more of an open book. Coaches get paid and get better jobs according to their records. No one seems inclined to be cheerful with regard to a coach whose athletes are not successful, even if they happen to have been cheated out of the results they deserve. Too many coaches took the path of least resistance when faced with that fact of life and resorted to copying the conduct they ought to have despised and brought to the attention of the sport and public authorities. Coaches are a major part of the problem.

Parents are the most complex riddle. Sometimes they want their children to succeed so badly that they disregard their health and psychological well-being. Sometimes they cease to draw a line between what they want and what their children want and they live a parallel life of success through their children's success. They become combatants themselves, fighting with other parents and even the sport officials or coaches for imagined errors or slights. They become obsessed with the sport careers of their children. They cease being responsible, balanced parents and become more childlike than their children. What a sad state of affairs!

STEP 4: EDUCATE EVERYBODY

In the long run, the solution requires a change of attitude away from the culture of doping and towards one that acknowledges that drug use in sport is wrong. This, in turn, requires a broad-based educational program that is directed at athletes, coaches and trainers, parents, physicians and the public in general. They have to understand the dangers involved where drugs are used in sport. And they have to insist—collectively and firmly—that ethical and medical standards be observed.

Is There a Cure? My Ten-Step Program

I do not want to minimize the difficulties that we face in such an effort, but we must persist in the effort until we are successful. The difficulties are compounded by ethical erosion in many aspects of society in general, including business, political and professional standards, academic cheating and a host of others. Sport is by no means alone in its ethical struggle, but it has its own responsibilities and will have no one to blame but itself if it allows its own ethical values to erode further. We are playing "catch up" with the cheaters. That is the price we pay for having allowed the situation to degenerate to the extent it already has.

The ultimate answer to doping in sport is education, not punishments. Don't get me wrong. We need the penalties as part of the arsenal in the fight against doping, but, in the end, it is only a small part of the cure. We need to concentrate on preventing doping in the first place, instead of just detecting it once it has already happened and punishing it. Part of the education will consist of making everyone aware that when doping occurs, it *will* be detected and penalties *will* follow. Realistically, I realize that some will stop using prohibitive drugs only because they are afraid of getting caught. While I would much rather that we could win their hearts and minds, in the final analysis, so long as the competitions are not tainted with cheating and young athletes' health is not being endangered, I could be relatively satisfied.

Educational programs must be directed at all levels of sport and in the communities where sport is practiced. We need to use all of the many channels of communication that exist today, including the web-based media, through which so many people can be reached at astonishingly low cost. We have already worked with the European Community on such programs in all of the 11 languages used in that continental grouping. We make educational programs available to countries that have never had the opportunity or capacity to develop their own. We have an athlete outreach program that puts us in direct contact with athletes at major events, so they understand the ramifications of doping and learn where they can find the information that will answer any questions. We encourage national anti-doping organizations to establish resources to answer questions or to create a help desk to respond to queries. Program modules are developed and made available to teachers for school use. I speak on many occasions to different groups, ranging from international conferences to small gatherings of Boy Scouts, from university settings to community groups, to business organizations, armed services and senior public servants to give them personal contact with the subject matter. I work hard at trying to engage them, since that is more powerful than merely having an intellectual understanding of the problem. I have never had someone reply "yes" when I ask if they want their children to be forced to use drugs in order to be successful in sport. I have never encountered anything but disgust when I describe some of the devices that are used to try to manipulate urine tests. The phenomenon of doping is so widespread, and the passive acceptance of it so profound, that it requires concerted and coordinated understanding and action for the cure to be effective. It is not enough to focus solely on the athletes, although they will obviously be a key audience.

STEP 5: ENSURE THAT THE RULES ARE FOLLOWED

I believe in the concept of the presumption of innocence. It is one of the cornerstones of our legal system. So, when athletes shows up for competition, it should be understood that they have agreed to follow the rules, including those against doping. On the other hand, based on past experience, it would be hopelessly naive to believe that every athlete would tell the truth. There have been just too many cases of cheaters lying to cover up their misdeeds. Athletes have repeatedly lied about everything from their ages to their genders and, of course, their doping activities. They are assisted in these lies by sports officials and doctors. So, while they are entitled to a presumption of innocence, they are also required by the rules of the sport to be tested to see whether they do comply. If they break a rule, they have every opportunity to know what the charges are and to be able to defend themselves.

It is not unlike the old Cold War adage of "trust, but verify." Generally, athletes who do not cheat do not object to these tests. The tests may be annoying, but they have a purpose that all of the athletes, innocent and guilty, understand. I suppose a parallel may be the cumbersome and time-consuming security checks we endure in airports. We recognize that these are necessary to fight the terrorist threat. While these security checks are irritating, it is nevertheless reassuring that everyone who gets on my plane has been subjected to the same search. The real hope—for all benign passengers and all clean athletes—is not for the tests to disappear, but rather that they instead be conducted with every possible state-of-the-art method and technology.

STEP 6: ELIMINATE CHEATERS

This is not a complicated concept. If you cheat, you are breaking the rules we have all agreed upon, and we don't want you around. If you don't agree with the rules, don't play. If you are in the competition and you cheat, you have spoiled it for everyone, including yourself, even if you may not be willing to recognize it. There is no reason why the rest of us should have to put up with your behavior or be forced to copy it just because you refuse to honor the promise you made when you entered the competition. The problem should be yours, not ours.

If you are someone who has helped an athlete to cheat, we don't want you anywhere near the sport or other athletes, for as long as possible. If you are supplying drugs to athletes, I hope you become acquainted with the police and the criminal justice system. If you are a doctor doing the same thing, I hope you lose your license to practice medicine. You have failed to observe the standards of a profession whose calling is to cure illness and to do no harm. If you are a sports official complicit in this kind of behavior, you should be booted out of office. When you think of it, there are precious few gray areas in doping. Most of it is pretty clearly black and white. Beware those who attempt to blur the lines.

STEP 7: RESEARCH

I often go to conferences about doping in sport. Two of the main arguments against anti-doping programs are that athletes should be able to do whatever they want, and that there can be no technological solution to doping so the effort should be abandoned as hopeless. The cheaters, they say, will always be ahead. As you close one loophole, the cheaters will find another, and the game will continue without end. I agree entirely, as I have said before, that the complete solution will not be technical, just as it will not be derived from punishing cheaters. I do not think that the situation is hopeless. It is an ongoing struggle, one without end, but better understanding of the drugs and methods used for doping and the development of better and more sophisticated tests are important functions in the overall fight against doping in sport. The knowledge gained helps in the educational efforts, and more data become available from athletes who have doped or been subjected to doping. And, of course, this knowledge makes it easier to enforce the rules.

WADA is now able to provide research funds for specialized investigation into doping science. Most sport organizations, at least those outside the profitable professional leagues, lived from hand to mouth and had no funds for research or testing. The WADA funding is significant, although much less than I would like to be able to contribute. On the other hand, the types of performance-enhancing drugs and methods are fairly limited. There are stimulants, anabolic steroids and similar substances, growth enhancers, oxygen enhancers, masking agents (to disguise the presence of prohibited substances), blood manipulation methods and a few others, plus, of course, gene doping. Research can be targeted in those areas where we understand that the abuses occur, and I am optimistic that the margin of maneuver for the cheaters who are using the substances and methods is being narrowed significantly and can continue to be narrowed. The wide road previously available for dopers has shrunk to a sidewalk and will shrink further to a balance beam and, eventually, to a tightrope—with no safety net.

STEP 8: FIND INTERNATIONAL SOLUTIONS

I cannot overemphasize the importance of a unified approach to the solution of doping in sport. Doping is not a local problem. It exists throughout the world and has to be treated as a global affliction, requiring a global treatment. There cannot be different rules for American or Canadian or Japanese or Indian or Russian athletes. They

CHAPTER FOURTEEN

all compete together in world events, such as the Olympics or world championships, and none of them should be able to claim special treatment. Huge progress has been achieved in the past five years in establishing this principle. The World Anti-Doping Code and its related standards have created a harmonized set of anti-doping rules for the sports movement. Adoption of the International Convention against Doping in Sport at the end of 2005 and its ratification and coming into force in 2006 have brought governments to the assistance of the sports movement by agreeing to implement the same rules as are contained in the Code, to eliminate the many differences between domestic and international sport legislation.

There will always be some difference of opinion about doping in sport, both as to what it means and what should be the consequences if it occurs. When we put the Code together, we had to reconcile widely differing approaches and the only solution was to find some consensus that everyone could accept, even if it meant that there were some misgivings about certain of the provisions. I personally favored penalties for a serious doping offence of more than two years, but there were many sport organizations that thought this would be too severe. Also, many governments thought that their state courts might decide to intervene if the penalties were longer than two years. So, we ended up with two years. This is a decision that can be reviewed periodically and it may well be that when the public comes to understand the impact of doping on all aspects of sport within the world community, there might be some possibility of change. In the short term, however, it was far more important to get some agreement on at least minimum standards than to hold out for some "perfect" solution.

The next step is to make sure that all of the stakeholders are actually implementing the Code. It is one thing to pay lip service to the concept, and quite another to put it into practice—since, when all is said and done, often more is said than done. WADA's role is to monitor compliance with the Code and to report on a regular basis. WADA does not have the jurisdiction to do more than to report; the power to act rests with the particular stakeholders, whether sport organizations or governments. I am looking forward to the first occasion on which we may have to report on non-compliance, not because I am vindictive, but because it will be a test of the resolve of the stakeholder to take the necessary steps to demonstrate that it means business. Make no mistake about it; there will be those who will push this to the very limit in the expectation that the sport or government authorities will not have the courage of their expressed opinions.

STEP 9: SEEK PARTNERS

There are many possible allies who can be encouraged to help in the fight against doping in sport, and we must take every opportunity to enlist that support. The most obvious source of allies can be found within sport itself. The vast majority of athletes, coaches and officials are involved in sport for the right reasons. They understand the importance of clean sport. They can speak out in a variety of ways—in interviews, in clinics, in practices, in op-ed articles, in letters to the editor, all of which will help create additional traction. Above all, they can set examples through their behavior. Someone once said, "What you do is so loud that I cannot hear what you say." You have to live the life for which you argue.

Even outside the confines of sport itself, there are many others who can be helpful. Legislators need to be urged to act. They rarely take the initiative, but they do respond

CHAPTER FOURTEEN

to pressure. Find people who can create that pressure. Community leaders can create pressure. Business leaders can create pressure. The public at large can create pressure, perhaps as much pressure as will be necessary, provided there can be enough education that "reaches" them and leads to a change in attitude. If you don't have the attitude, it will never become a cause. The 2005 U.S. congressional hearings on doping in sport came about as a result of pressure and, once underway, such processes can achieve results, even if they fall short of legislation. Doctors can generate pressure by professing the health risks of doping. Parents can create pressure, and if they have a tale to tell about a child injured or killed because of drug use, the public at large and legislators as well will listen.

Just as sponsors were influential in helping to create some changes within the IOC following the Salt Lake City bidding scandal, they could be influential in the fight against doping in sport. They could withhold support from federations or national Olympic committees that do not have effective anti-doping programs. They could withhold support from Olympic organizing committees and the IOC if the Code is not properly applied. They could stop supporting, through advertising or ticket purchases, professional leagues that do not have vigorous anti-doping programs. They can understand the damage caused to their own brands if the sport franchises they happen to support are willing to turn a blind eye to cheating. Quite apart from whatever their own ethical feelings may be about cheating in sport, if their brands are damaged by association with cheating, their stewardship of corporate resources will be inadequate. Write your company president if you see this occurring. You, too, can create pressure.

If you are a public official, especially one who is elected, there are many things you can do to help stop doping in sport. You can cut off public funding, whether direct or indirect, to organizations that do not implement effective anti-doping programs. You can pay attention to your constituents or even your own conscience as a public servant. The same should be true for athletes who test positive and for coaches and other officials who are involved with that doping. Legislators can adopt laws or regulations that would deny access by any organization not implementing an effective anti-doping program to any facility that has had a single dollar of financial assistance provided by the public. No facilities should receive any public funding unless the tenants and any teams they play adopt such anti-doping programs. Money spent on sports or teams without anti-doping programs should not get tax deductions. Why should the public support luxury boxes used to watch doped-up athletes? Governments should do whatever they can to ratify the International Anti-Doping Convention adopted at the UNESCO General Conference in 2005 and then take the necessary steps to incorporate the World Anti-Doping Code as part of their domestic law. These are all actions that legislators, whether at the grass roots or at the summit of political power, can do on their own. And they should do this on their own. And if not on their own, for the right reasons, then in their own self-interests, as a program to get re-elected. Would it not be a welcome change to have done something good without being forced to do so?

STEP 10: NEVER GIVE UP—IT'S TOO IMPORTANT

Many credit Winston Churchill with saving Great Britain during World War II. One of his best-known morale-building speeches was given in October 1941, when the outcome of the war was still very much in doubt. What he

CHAPTER FOURTEEN

said expresses the attitude that must prevail in order to win sport's world war against doping: "Never give in, never give in, never, never, never—in nothing, great or small, large or petty—never give in except to convictions of honour and good sense."

It is my current lot in life that I have been designated as the President of WADA. I am not unhappy with the idea, because I do think that doping in sport is the principal challenge that will be faced by sport in the next few years. I do not think that responsible parents want their children to have to become dopers in order to be successful in sport. If the situation is not brought under control, they may well discourage their children from going into competitive sport. If that happens often enough, the future of sport may be in doubt.

Strong action is required and I will have no hesitation in using the powers of WADA to help stamp out cheating in sport. Our aim is to protect those who compete fairly. Prevention is the long-term key. In the interim, there must be effective enforcement of the rules.

As many can attest, I am no diplomat. I do not think you have to tiptoe around the fact that people are cheating. I believe that they should be caught, identified and taken out of the competitions. It is also important to identify those who help athletes to cheat, and those who force them to cheat, and those who allow them to cheat.

In my view, nothing can justify such behavior, and I will do everything in my power to make sure that the enablers, along with the guilty athletes, are exposed and punished. We will enlist the public in our fight. This is a war that we simply cannot afford to lose. The future of sport and of our children depend on it.

AFTERWORD

I always knew it would be risky to try to do a book on doping and the fight to keep sport clean because there are new developments every day. That is why I tried to illustrate many of the points I was trying to make with examples. In fact, probably the ideal means of publishing a book like this would be to use an interactive format that could be updated on a daily or hourly basis! Two cases in point arose after the book had gone to publication, indeed after I had reviewed page proofs—the final step before it is bound and printed.

TOUR TROUBLES

One was the 2006 Tour de France, the first in the post–Lance Armstrong era. The Tour got off to a rocky start with the revelations arising from a comprehensive investigation by the Spanish authorities. After investigating, interviewing witnesses, seizing documents and observing the behavior of athletes and their entourages, Spanish authorities concluded that there

AFTERWORD

was an organized conspiracy. This was announced shortly before the start of the Tour, but, initially, no names were disclosed, which was normal procedure in Spain. Because many of the riders implicated in the investigation would be competing in the Tour, the Spanish authorities decided that they would advise the International Cycling Union (UCI) in advance of the race so that it could decide whether or not it should take any action. The UCI did not make the names public, but advised the teams for which the riders competed. The teams announced the names of the athletes and declared that they would be prevented from participating in the 2006 Tour.

This news of a doping conspiracy was bad enough as a general blot on cycling, but when the names were released, they included the riders who had finished second, third, fourth, fifth and sixth in the 2005 Tour! This was not simply an isolated example of a single rider here and there who had been implicated. Nor was it limited to riders at the back of the peleton, possibly using drugs to try to keep up with the leaders. No, it was the leaders themselves, the presumptive heirs to the recently retired Armstrong. The list also included Tyler Hamilton, whose "vanishing twin" appeared to have been replaced by a regimen of drugs prescribed by a Spanish doctor, and dozens of other riders. Even a UCI official was implicated in the activities. It could not have been worse for cycling and the UCI, which, as recently as April 2006, had assured me and other WADA officials that there had been a complete attitude change in the sport and that the UCI was considering a reduction in the number of tests, since they were no longer dealing with a widespread doping problem in the sport. Interest in the 2006 Tour was greatly diminished, partly because of the absence of the anticipated new generation of stars and partly because it was finally beginning to dawn on the public that little, if any, progress had been made in

AFTERWORD

cleaning up the sport since the Festina scandal in 1998. The tacit acceptance of some doping in the sport had allowed the virus to spread, and it now appeared that the successors to Armstrong had been identified with doping practices. It was worse than I had feared, and I am no great admirer of cycling's effectiveness in dealing with doping.

The diminished Tour ran its course, desperately seeking a new hero, and it appeared that its prayers may have been answered in the person of Floyd Landis, an American rider with the Phonak team. He had been in and around the lead on a number of occasions during the race but had fallen well behind at one stage and was considered to be out of the running until he staged a miracle comeback in one of the difficult mountain stages, an almost unheard-of feat that was the subject of universal admiration for courage and determination in the face of overwhelming odds. Landis went on to win the Tour. It gave the Tour a much-needed shot in the arm. Perhaps the future was not as black as it had seemed, and the cycling fraternity must have breathed a sigh of relief. The ongoing Spanish affair would unfold over time, but that would be months or years, given the delays inherent in the criminal justice system. For now, however, there was a new hero in the Tour de France, an unlikely former journeyman—a rags-to-riches scenario—that could be a tale for the ages.

Except for one thing...

DEFROCKED NEW HERO

On the Thursday following Landis's tumultuous entry into Paris and the ceremonial lap around the Arc de Triomphe accorded to the winner of the Tour de France, a brief announcement was made by the UCI that a rider in the Tour had been found to have a prohibited substance in his system. Details were provided to the rider's team. Shortly thereafter, Phonak announced that the rider was Landis and that the laboratory had detected elevated levels of testosterone in the urine provided by Landis in the course of a doping control. The test in question was one taken on the day of the astonishing comeback staged by Landis. Phonak also said that it had suspended Landis from any further competitions pending resolution of the matter. As happens in 99.99% of the cases, Landis denied that he had used any performance-enhancing substance and called for analysis of the second, or "B" sample, to see if that would confirm the analysis of the first sample. If the analysis of the "B" sample did not confirm the "A" sample, there would be no doping offence and he would remain champion of the 2006 Tour de France. But, if it did, he would be in deep trouble. Testing for elevated testosterone is based essentially on the ratio between testosterone and epitestosterone in the body. In normal people that ratio is 1:1 and might go as high, in unusual cases, as 2:1. In order to be careful not to have false positive tests, the sports movement (as reflected in the List prepared for purposes of the World Anti-Doping Code) has set a ratio of 4:1, to provide ample room to absorb extremely unusual cases of high testosterone produced naturally. The ratio used to be 6:1, but it transpired that athletes were deliberately using testosterone and keeping their levels just under the 6:1 ratio, so it was lowered to the present 4:1. Landis's sample registered a ratio of 11:1—almost three times the allowable level and approximately ten times the normal level!

There was little doubt that the "B" sample analysis would confirm the first analysis. Even Landis acknowledged that it probably would. On August 5, the UCI announced, to no one's surprise, that the "B" sample was also positive for elevated testosterone levels. It also noted that the level

AFTERWORD

involved was a ratio of 11:1. In the interim, Landis and his entourage offered several explanations for the result of the "A" sample. These included the fairly standard suggestion that he had naturally high testosterone levels. This had not generated much traction, since he had been tested on other occasions during the same Tour (and many occasions prior to the 2006 event) and, if the condition had been natural, there would have been a record of it, to which he could easily have pointed. Other suggestions were that he had used glucocortico steroids for a hip condition and some medication for a thyroid condition, none of which, in fact, would have had an impact on testosterone production or levels. He then speculated that it might have been a result of a beer he had consumed, or some whiskey. It sounded like he might have taken a play from the unsuccessful Dennis Mitchell, who blamed his positive result on beer and sexual intercourse. None other than Lance Armstrong himself waded into the fray in support of Landis, in the course of which he noted, darkly, that the laboratory involved was the same IOC and now WADA-laboratory that had found traces of EPO in six of his 1999 Tour de France samples. Yes, it was indeed the same accredited laboratory. Armstrong did not, however, seem to realize that his statement cut both ways—that a credible finding of proper analytical procedures and standards in the Landis matter might well reinforce the credibility of the laboratory's EPO analyses of the 1999 samples. This statement, combined with the impact of the 2006 Tour disqualifications and the self-serving smokescreen thrown up by the discredited ICU-commissioned "independent" investigation, has done much to keep the controversy regarding Armstrong active.

So, instead of a shot in the arm for cycling, the ill-fated 2006 Tour has proved to have been a shot in the foot. Not only were the top riders from the 2005 Tour suspended, but

AFTERWORD

the winner of the 2006 Tour had tested positive. No one on the face of the planet could have any faith in what was going on in the races. What did it mean about past races? One of the German television networks, ZDF—and remember that cycling is extremely popular in Germany—announced that it might not cover the Tour any longer, since it had signed a broadcasting contract for a sporting event, not a show demonstrating the performance of the pharmaceutical industry. The UCI president solemnly announced that there would be a "crusade" against doping—the problem was now elevated from a "scourge" to be eliminated, to a fight to be pursued with religious fervor. Let's hope it will not be with horses and lances, but with all the tools available in a more modern world. Based on past performance, I do not think that the UCI is capable of doing this on its own, even if it were to make the changes in its testing programs that we suggested before these scandals broke. It has been far too concerned with trying to justify its actions, pointing to the number of tests that it performs and complaining about any criticism directed its way by others, including WADA and me. I think it will have to acknowledge that it needs help from international organizations like WADA and Interpol, as well as the public authorities, and from its sponsors, tour directors and broadcasters. Sports organizations do know who the athletes are, where they are, what they are likely to be using, who the coaches and trainers may be, who the suspect doctors may be; but they do not have the power to search for evidence, to require witnesses to give evidence, to seize incriminating materials. The days are long gone when the only way to prove a doping offence was by a positive analytical sample. Tackling sophisticated sport "criminals" requires the same sophisticated and integrated approach as dealing with standard criminals. For international federations to wrap themselves in their sacred autonomy is all but to guarantee that there will be no effective solution to doping in their sport. I hope that the UCI does not take such a myopic view of its current circumstances, or it may never recover.

PILING ON

As if all the cycling furor were not enough for the summer of 2006, during the same weekend when everyone was waiting for the confirmation of Landis's test came the announcement from the handlers of Justin Gatlin, the current Olympic champion, world champion and world record holder in the 100 meters, that he had tested positive for testosterone or its precursors. This was his second positive test, which means he faces the possibility of a lifetime suspension. He had served a sanction earlier for a prohibited substance, amphetamine, contained in Adderall, a medicine he said he was taking to deal with an attention deficit syndrome. On this occasion, there was no need to wait for the "B" analysis—that had all been done before his publicists had made the public announcement. The test had been performed at a competition in April, and the matter had been kept confidential for almost three months. The affair is now in the hands of the United States Anti-Doping Agency to consider the appropriate penalty, which will be reviewed by the IAAF and WADA, both of which, as well as Gatlin himself, have rights to appeal to the Court of Arbitration for Sport if the sanction given is not in accordance with the World Anti-Doping Code.

USADA says it will not comment on a case that is in progress. The USOC says it is clear that the fight against doping in sport is not over. USA Track and Field says it is concerned that someone like Gatlin, who has been a spokesperson for drug-free sport, has been caught, but hopes

AFTERWORD

that it will not be a doping offence and says that it does not matter who you are if you are caught doping. The IAAF has signaled that USADA should be looking at a lifetime ban. The agent of the co–world record holder, Asafa Powell says that a lifetime ban is too easy: doping cheaters should go to jail. Gatlin himself is unable to account for the positive test and denied ever having knowingly used the drugs or authorizing anyone to administer them to him. His coach, Trevor Graham, himself under grand jury investigation for possibly using drugs with his athletes, several of whom have been sanctioned for drug use (Graham denies any involvement), says that the sample was sabotaged and that he can prove who did it. It turns out that it was not the sample that was sabotaged, but that a masseur with a grudge had rubbed a tainted mixture on the athlete's legs. The masseur denies any such action.

The whole mess goes on and on, with spokespersons, agents, lawyers and publicists offering suggestions, defenses, excuses, theories of varying complexity, pseudo-science and more or less fanciful explanations. One feature of the whole doping phenomenon is the frighteningly small number of athletes and others who are prepared to acknowledge that they have, in fact, doped or helped to dope. Denial is the watchword and it is repeated like a mantra, not that it will persuade anyone these days, especially when the evidence is overwhelming as to what has happened. Probably as a result of "lawyering," many of the athletes are moving away from the absolute blanket denial to say that they have never "knowingly" taken prohibited substances. However, it does not matter whether they were taken knowingly or not—if they were found in the athlete's system, that is all that matters. Oh yes, and there will always be the statement that the athlete has never tested positive in the past. It would be almost refreshing for someone who has been caught to say that the decision was correct, he or she had been doping and deserved the penalty that was imposed. At least they would deserve some respect for acknowledging their guilt and trying to move on. It is the pig-headed ones who are unwilling to face up to the consequences of their own acts for whom I have no sympathy whatsoever. In addition to being cheaters, they are cowards.

Here are two of the most important sports in the world whose marquis athletes have been identified as dopers. Whatever is being done is falling well short of dealing with the problem, and the long-term risks for the sports are extreme. Right now, I have no interest in watching the Tour de France or any other professional road race and am not even willing to tune in to such events on free television. I stopped going to the world athletics championships almost twenty years ago. I watch them during the Olympic Games because at the Games I know we are trying to do everything possible to have drug-free Games, but not otherwise. I doubt very much that I am alone and, what is worse, I am someone who loves sport and everything it has the potential to become. Imagine people who are ambivalent about sport in the first place, who might be willing to watch genuine sport but who have no interest whatsoever in some counterfeit version of the real thing. They will certainly vote with their feet—there are too many alternatives competing for their attention.

NEVER GIVE IN, NEVER...

This is a call to action—serious and concerted—by those who believe in sport. No matter who and where you are, speak out against cheating, against those who assist the cheaters and those responsible for sport who do not do everything in their power to fulfill their responsibilities.

AFTERWORD

Make an example of them and one of yourselves, so you can be proud of what is accomplished on the field of play. Or, soon, it may not matter. A class of professional, humanoid gladiators will take over an extreme entertainment business that has no other purpose and your greatest fear may be that one of your kids will be part of it.

INDEX

A
academia, 30
accidental use, 67–68
Adderall, 235
Afghanistan, 176
Agricola, Riccardo, 174
alcohol, 49, 50
Alzado, Lyle, 138
Amgen, 165
amphetamines, 133, 235
anabolic agents. *See* anabolic steroids
anabolic steroids
    about, 42–43
    acknowledgement of use, 138
    business of, 163
    deaths from use of, 26
    excuses for use, 80–81, 83
    illegal production of, 175
    MLB testing, 125
    sales figures, 166
    sources of, 172, 173
    trafficking of, 175
    users of, 175–177
anti-doping rules
    arguments against, 37–38
    origin of, 11
    variations in, 93, 94–96, 111–112
    See also UNESCO International Convention Against Doping in Sport; World Anti-Doping Code
anti-oestrogenic agents, 45
Arabian Gulf, 175
Arbeit, Ekkart, 114
Armstrong, Lance
    chairman of WADA and, 94, 150
    EPO use allegations, 190–194
    support of Landis, 233
    in Tour de France, 69
    TV shows, 195–197
    UCI investigation, 197–201

artificial oxygen carriers, 46
Association of Tennis Players (ATP), 82, 158
asthma, 207
Athens Summer Olympics (2004), 92, 143
athletes
    attitude of, 118–120
    awareness of doping, 203–205
    compliance with rules, 106–107, 215–216, 220–221
    effect of cheating, 13–14
    influence of, 175, 176–177
    motivations of, 216–217
    public awareness of drug use, 209
    reporting drug use, 20–21, 203–205
    See also professional sports
Atlanta Summer Olympics (1996), 68–69
ATP (Association of Tennis Players), 82, 158
attitude
    of athletes, 118–120
    change through education, 218–220
    of general public, 1, 209–211
Australian Rules football, 41
Austria, 75
Austrian cross-country skiing team, 72–75, 81
Austrian Olympic Committee, 75, 77
Austrian ski federation, 72, 75

B
Baggaley, Nathan, 81, 84
Balco scandal, 25, 57–61, 85–89, 205
Banned List
    gene doping, 184–185
    prohibited substances and methods, 42–46, 47–50
    removing substances or methods, 215
    yearly updating, 40–42, 101–102

INDEX

Barcelona Summer Olympics (1992), 142–143
baseball
 cheating in, 20
 deaths, 4
 international federation, 131
 See also MLB (Major League Baseball)
Baseball Hall of Fame, 132
basketball, 141–144, 182
Baumann, Dieter, 80
Bechler, Steve, 4, 124
Beijing Summer Olympics (2008), 180
benzedrine, 176
Berard, Brian, 149
beta-blockers, 49, 50, 157
beta-2 agonists, 44–45, 50, 207
Bettman, Gary, 149–150
biathlon, 69, 72–75
Blatter, Joseph, 154
blood doping
 about, 45–46
 excuses for, 81
 international meeting, 71
 investigation of use, 72–75
Bonds, Barry, 20, 38, 81–82, 109, 132, 135, 161
boxing, 158
bromantan, 68–69
Bush, George W., 127–128

C

Caborn, Richard, 169
Canada
 anti-doping policy, 62
 drug use laws, 76
 UNESCO convention, 102
Canadian Football League (CFL), 68, 140
cannabinoids, 48, 50
Canseco, José, 38, 124
Carolina Panthers, 69, 207
CAS (Court of Arbitration for Sport)
 Baggaley ruling, 81
 FIFA anti-doping and, 155–156
 Lund case, 82–83
 Montgomery case, 87–88
 professional sports and, 160
 responsibilities of, 101
 view on penalties, 112
catheters, 46, 68, 85

CBS television network, 31–32
Ceriani, Marco, 4
CFL (Canadian Football League), 68, 140
Chambers, Dwain, 113
cheating
 as breach of rules, 106
 doping as, 15, 37
 effect on sports, 110
 gaining advantage, 19–20, 215–216
 motivations for, 9, 12
 prevention of, 13, 221–222, 237–238
chemical manipulation of urine, 46
China
 doping in, 25, 62–63
 drug manufacturers, 169–170
 steroid exports, 175
 systemized programs, 69, 206
Christie, Linford, 95–96
Churchill, Winston, 227–228
clenbuterol, 83
cloning scandal, 30
coaches
 awareness of doping, 63–64
 importance of winning, 27
 motivations of, 218
 rationalizations, 214
 responsibilities of, 23–24, 120, 205–207
 right to coach, 114
 role of, 14–15, 22
 as source of doping, 61
cocaine, 80, 83, 163, 173
Collins, Michelle, 59
compliance, monitoring, 103
 See also rules
compulsory testing, 108
confidentiality, 107
Conte, Victor, 25, 58–61, 86, 88
Copenhagen Declaration, 98
corticosteroids, 48–50
corticotrophins, 43, 44
Costas, Bob, 195–196
Court of Arbitration for Sport (CAS). See CAS
cricket, 41, 158
cross-country skiing
 blood doping, 72–75
 drug testing, 69, 204
 EPO use in, 165

INDEX

cycling
    adoption of code, 101
    deaths, 4
    drug use in, 201–202
    EPO use in, 65, 165, 166–167, 190–194
    hematocrit level in, 70
    opportunities for manipulation, 85
    systemized programs, 69
    See also Spain doping investigation

D

Daly, Bill, 150
de Villiers, Pieter, 83
DEA (US Drug Enforcement Agency), 172–173
deaths, 4, 26, 36, 56, 121, 124, 137
denial, 214, 236–237
Di Tomasso, David, 4
dilution, 85
distribution. *See* trafficking
diuretics, 45, 80–81, 83
doctors
    assistance in cover-ups, 221
    codes of conduct for, 117–118
    convictions of, 174, 207
    effect of cheating, 14
    penalties for supplying, 170, 171
    pressuring for change, 226
    rationalizations, 214
    responsibilities of, 114–117, 207–208
doping
    co-conspirators in, 12–13
    convictions, 87–89
    defined, 11
    eliminating, 213–214
    escalating, 21
    excuses for, 80–84
    initiation to, 63
    as offence, 16
    proof of, 86–89, 107
    risks of, 3–4, 36–37
    systemized programs, 20, 68–69
    timing of use, 85
    widespread use of, 54–55
doping control forms
    in EPO use allegations, 191–192
    modifications to, 15
doping rules. *See* anti-doping rules; UNESCO International Convention Against Doping in Sport; World Anti-Doping Code
Dream Team, 142–143
drugs
    availability of, 2
    dangers of allowing use, 1
    prohibited, 42–46, 47–50
    See also doping

E

East Germany
    acceptance of doping, 25
    coaches, 62, 114, 206
    doctors, 208
    systemized doping programs, 20, 52–54
Eastern Europe, 173
ecstasy, 83
education, 120, 218–220
Edwards, Paul, 83
Ender, Kornelia, 54
endurance sports, 165
enforcement
    of existing laws, 76
    improvements to, 37–38
    in professional sports, 159–161, 211
    role of WADA, 92–94, 228
    by sports federations, 96
enthusiasm, 28
ephedrine, 50, 124
epitestosterone, 46, 232
EPO (erythropoietin)
    about, 43
    in cycling, 65, 165, 190–203
    excuses for using, 83
    need for testing, 71
    possession of, 166–167
    testing, 60
    therapeutic uses of, 164–165
    in track and field, 58
    worldwide sales, 164, 165
estrogen, 45
ethics
    allowing drug use and, 2
    erosion of values, 29, 219
    in gene doping, 187–188
    of medical profession, 115–116, 208
    need for understanding of, 120

INDEX

in Olympic Movement, 10–11
of pharmaceutical companies, 117
value of, 7
European Community, 219
evidence other than positive test, 86–89
Ewald, Manfred, 53–54
excuses, 80–84, 236–237
experimentation on athletes, 64–65
exposure of doping, 92

F

facilities, 227
Fauviau, Christoph, 25–26
Feher, Miklos, 4
Fehr, Don, 135
Ferrari, Michele, 174, 193
Festina team, 91–92, 166, 191, 202
FIBA (Fédération Internationale de Basketball), 142–143
FIFA (Fédération Internationale de Football Association), 152–156
figure skating, 14
finasteride, 41, 82
Finchem, Tim, 157–158
FIS (International Ski Federation), 71, 72
Foe, Marc-Vivien, 4
football. *See* NFL (National Football League)
football, Australian Rules, 41
France
 laws in, 166–167, 174
 resentment of Tour de France winners, 197
Francis, Charlie, 24–25, 64, 114
French Cycling Federation, 92
Friedmann, Ted, 182
furosemide, 83

G

Gaines, Chrystie, 205
Galetti, Alessio, 4
gambling, 132
Gate, George, 23
Gatlin, Justin, 235–236
Gavrilova, Anzhelika, 83
gene doping
 about, 2, 46, 179–181
 concerns with, 181–183
 ethics of, 187–188

regulating, 183
testing for, 184–186
generic drugs, 166, 169–170
genetics, cloning scandal, 30
German Democratic Republic. *See* East Germany
Germany, 186, 206
Giro d'Italia, 167
glucocorticosteroids, 48–50
Goldman, Brian, 60
golf, 157–158
gonadotrophins (hCG), 43, 44
Goodenow, Bob, 145
governments
 adoption of code, 99
 international convention on doping, 101
 pressuring for change, 225–227
 regulation of drug distribution, 170–171
 responsibilities of, 103, 160
 support of code, 98
 support of independent agency, 92–93
 trafficking penalties, 172–173, 177
 winning and, 53–54
Graham, Trevor, 236
Greek athletics federation, 92
Grimsley, Jason, 109
growth hormone. *See* hGH (human growth hormone)

H

Hamilton, Tyler, 81, 230
hash, 48
hCG (human chorionic gonadotrophin), 43, 44
health test, 69–70
heart attack deaths, 4, 36, 56
hematocrit level, 69–70
heroin, 47–48, 163, 173
hGH (human growth hormone)
 about, 43–44
 excuses for using, 83
 possession of, 166–167
 potential for use, 142
 problems in testing for, 85
 testing development, 87–88
 worldwide sales, 165

INDEX

historical data, 71
hockey, 99, 145–152
Hooton, Taylor, 26
hormones, 43–44
  See also specific hormones
horse racing, 158
human chorionic gonadotrophin (hCG), 43, 44
human growth hormone. *See* hGH (human growth hormone)
Hunter, C.J., 83

I

IAAF (International Association of Athletics Federations)
  Chambers case, 113
  Gatlin case, 235–236
  White case, 56–57
IFs (international federations)
  adoption of code, 100–101
  involvement in code development, 97–98
  variations in doping rules, 96, 111–112
  view on penalties, 112
IIHF (International Ice Hockey Federation), 99, 150–151
India
  doping in, 63
  drug manufacturers, 169–170
  steroid exports, 175
Inoue, Junsuke, 83
insulin, 43, 44
International Association of Athletics Federations (IAAF). *See* IAAF
international basketball federation (FIBA), 142–143
International Cycling Union. *See* UCI (Union Cycliste Internationale)
international federations. *See* IFs (international federations)
International Ice Hockey Federation (IIHF), 99, 150–151
International Ski Federation (FIS), 71, 72
International soccer federation (FIFA), 152–156
International Tennis Federation (ITF), 158
Internet, 177

Interpol, 165, 172–173, 234
IOC (International Olympic Committee)
  adoption of code, 99–100
  Austrian ski investigation, 72–77
  doping policies, 78, 91–92, 93
  drug list, 40
  removal of baseball, 130–131
  support of code, 97
IOC Athletes' Commission, 15
Iraq, 175, 176
Ismaili Muslims, 176
Italy
  drug laws, 75–77, 174
  police investigations, 73–75, 206
  trafficking in, 175

J

Jimenez, Jose Maria, 4
Johnson, Ben, 24, 62, 96, 115–116
Johnson & Johnson, 165
Jones, Marion, 86, 88, 114
Juventus, 174

K

Karatantcheva, Sesil, 82
Kennedy, John F., 78
Kenteris, Konstantinos, 92
Kirin, 165
Korchemny, Remi, 25, 58–61, 86
Kuwait, 175

L

Landis, Floyd, 231–233
Larry King Live, 195–196
laws, 75–78, 166–167, 174
lawyers, 105, 107, 108
LeMond, Greg, 197
L'Equipe, 190–191, 197–198, 199
Lincoln, Abraham, 103
Lombardi, Vince, 27, 28, 210
longitudinal follow-ups, 71
Lund, Zack, 82, 84, 113

M

Ma Junren, 83
Major League Baseball (MLB). *See* MLB
marijuana, 48, 163, 173
markers, 164–165
masking agents

243

INDEX

defined, 40–41
excuses for use, 80–81, 82, 83
function of, 45, 85
in track and field, 58
Mayer, Walter, 72–75
McCain, John, 130
McGwire, Mark, 20, 38, 109, 132, 135
McQuaid, Pat, 202
media
    access to professional sports, 123–124
    Armstrong EPO use allegations, 190–191, 195–197
    educational programs through, 219
    future cycling broadcasts, 234
    ratings, 211
    scandals in, 31–32
    view of NHL doping, 151
medical associations. *See* professional associations
Merck Vioxx, 30
methadone, 47–48
methytestosterone, 83
military, 175, 176
Miller, Bode, 108
Mitchell, Dennis, 80
Mitchell, George, 136
MLB (Major League Baseball)
    agreement to rules of sport, 110
    attitude of, 137, 144
    effect of attitude to doping, 129, 130–132
    on gambling, 132
    investigation of doping allegations, 136
    penalties for drug use, 109, 126, 133
    testing, 124–125, 133–134
MLBPA (Major League Baseball Players Association), 126, 134–135
modafinil, 56–61
money
    the business of professional sports, 161
    as motivation, 61, 177, 216–217
    return of, 113
Montgomery, Tim, 86–89, 114, 205
morphine, 47–48
motivations, 61, 216–217
Munich Summer Olympics (1972), 53

N

nandrolone, 80, 82
narcotics, 47–48
National Basketball Association (NBA), 141–144
national federations, 96
National Football League (NFL). *See* NFL
National Hockey League (NHL), 99, 145–152
National Hockey League Players Association, 145–146, 148, 151–152
National Institute of Health (NIH) Recombinant DNA Advisory Committee, 182
National Olympic committees (NOCs). *See* NOCs
NBA (National Basketball Association), 141–144
NFL (National Football League)
    doping in, 137–141
    as entertainment, 209–210
    penalties, 68, 144
    systemized programs, 69, 207
NHL (National Hockey League), 99, 145–152
NHLPA (Players Association), 145–146, 148, 151–152
"no fault" ruling, 112–113
no "significant" fault ruling, 113
NOCs (National Olympic committees)
    adoption of code, 100–101
    doping enforcement variations, 96
Norman, Greg, 157

O

Ocean Falls, BC, 22–23
oestrogen, 45
officials
    assistance in cover-ups, 221
    criticism of efforts, 204
    effect of cheating, 13–14
    rationalizations, 214
Olympic Games
    NHL player testing, 150–151
    soccer in, 153, 156
    See also specific Games
Olympics
    Charter, 99–100
    outreach programs, 120
    value of, 10

INDEX

See also IOC (International Olympic Committee)
organized crime, 163, 167, 175
out-of-competition testing, 71, 72–73, 94
outreach programs, 120, 220
oxygen transfer enhancement, 45–46

P
Palmeiro, Rafael, 79–80, 109, 132
Pantani, Marco, 4
parents
    attitude of, 25–26
    motivations of, 218
    responsibilities of, 120, 226
Paris World Championships (2003), 56–57
patient autonomy, 115–117
Pelletier, David, 14
penalties
    length of, 224
    in MLB, 133
    need for, 219, 221–222
    World Anti-Doping Code and, 111–113
penises, artificial, 68
performance-enhancing substances and methods. *See* doping; *specific drugs and methods*
Perth World Swimming Championships (1998), 62
Pfizer Inc., 168
PGA (Professional Golfers' Association), 157–158
pharmaceutical companies
    collaboration with WADA, 167–169
    ethics of, 29–30, 117
    worldwide sales, 164, 165–166
pharmacological manipulation of urine, 46
Phonak team, 231–233
physical manipulation of urine, 46
physicians. *See* doctors
pilots, 176
plagiarism, 30
police
    investigations of drug use, 73–75, 92
    use of drugs, 176
positive test, lack of, 84–89
possession, 77, 88

prescription audits, 170–171
Price, Nick, 157
probenicid, 50
production of drugs, 164–170
professional associations
    ethical rule enforcement, 116–117, 208
    penalizing suppliers, 171
professional sports
    Balco scandal, 86
    as a business, 122–123, 209–211
    drug use attitudes, 159–162
    government response to doping practices, 127–128
    influence of athletes, 27, 38
    objective of, 121
    support of WADA, 94
    World Anti-Doping Code and, 41
prohibited substances. *See* Banned List
proof, lack of, 84–89
pseudoephedrine, 115
Puerta, Mariano, 81
punishment. *See* penalties

R
Raducan, Andrea, 115
Rather, Dan, 31
rationalizations, 214
recognition, 217
recreational drugs, 141–142
red blood cell levels, 69–70
Reinholds, Andris, 83
religion, 32
reporting drug use, 20–21, 203–205, 237–238
Repoxygen, 186
research, 168, 222–223
respect, 237
Reynolds, Butch, 233
Roche, 165
Rogge, Jacques, 74–75, 199, 201
role models, 1, 27, 38
Romanowski, Bill, 138
Rose, Pete, 132
rowing, 95
rugby, 158
rules
    agreement to play by, 106–108, 110, 215–216, 220–221

245

INDEX

existence of in sports, 8–9, 38
importance of, 11
international, 223–225
variations in doping rules, 93, 94–96, 111–112
Rumsas, Edita, 166–167
Rumsas, Raimondas, 83, 166–167
running, 165
Rusconi, Marco, 4
Rusedski, Greg, 82
Russia, 175

S

Salanson, Fabrice, 4
salbutamol, 44–45
Salé, Jamie, 14
Salt Lake City Winter Olympics (2002)
    cross-country skiing, 72, 81, 204
    figure skating officials, 14
    report on scandal, 136
    sponsor pressure, 226
Samaranch, Juan Antonio
    interview with, 31–32
    view on doping, 91–92, 99–100
sanctions. *See* penalties
Sankyo, 165
Saskin, Ted, 150
Saturday Night Live, 196–197
scandals, 29–33
    See also Balco scandal; Festina team; Spain doping investigation
Schollander, Don, 27–28
Schüssel, Wolfgang, 74–75
scientists, 14
Scott, Beckie, 204–205
Selig, Bud, 136
Seoul Summer Olympics (1988), 24, 62
Sermon, Johan, 4
Sheen, Fulton, 16
shooting, 49
60 Minutes, 31–32
ski boot measurement, 108
Smith, Onterrio, 68
soccer
    deaths, 4
    in Italy, 206
    Juventus investigation, 174
    in Olympics, 152–153
    systemized programs, 69

World Anti-Doping Code and, 153–156
softball, 131–132
somatic cell modification, 180
soporifics, 176
Sosa, Sammy, 20, 132, 135
Sotomayor, Javier, 80
South Africa, 175
South America, 173
Soviet bloc
    acceptance of doping, 25
    systemized programs, 68–69
Spain doping investigation, 67, 69, 201, 202, 229–231
specified substances, 50
speed skating, 217
sponsors, 226
sports
    accepting rules, 106–108, 110, 215–216, 220–221
    importance of, 7–8, 28–29
    values in, 32–33
sports officials. *See* officials
sports organizations
    ability to fight doping, 234
    exposure of doping, 92
    responsibilities of, 189
    trafficking rules, 172
    variations in doping rules, 94–96
    See also IFs (international federations); *individual organizations*
sprinters, 165
stanozolol, 24
Stapleton, Bill, 192
State of the Union address, 127–128
Stern, David, 141
steroids. *See* anabolic steroids
stimulants
    about, 47
    MLB testing, 133
    use in military, 176
strict liability, 107
Sweden, 102
Sydney Summer Olympics (2000)
    basketball, 143
    WADA objectives for, 94

T

targeted testing, 70, 205

INDEX

temptations
   to coaches, 24
   to gain advantage, 21
tennis
   adoption of code, 158
   excuses for positive tests, 82
   in Olympic Games, 153
   World Anti-Doping Code and, 41
testing
   chaperones, 85
   compulsory, 108
   out-of-competition, 71, 72–73, 94
   targeted, 70, 205
testosterone
   about, 42–43
   in cycling, 232–233
   effect of hCG on, 44
   excuses for use, 80
   possession of, 166–167
   ratio for testing, 232
   sources of, 172
   in track and field, 235–236
   use in military, 176
Thanou, Ekaterini, 92
Théodore, José, 82, 149
therapeutic use exemptions (TUEs). *See* TUEs
THG
   lack of testing for, 14
   risks of, 65
   tip-off to, 64
   in track and field, 57–60, 85–87, 113
   See also Balco scandal
timing of use, 85
Tour de France
   adoption of code, 101
   EPO use allegations, 190
   Festina team scandal, 91–92, 166, 191, 202
   French resentment, 197
   Spanish doping investigation, 67, 69, 201, 202, 229–231
   2006 winner, 231–233
track and field
   EPO use in, 58, 165
   steroid use in, 115
   testosterone use in, 235–236
   THG use in, 85–87, 113
trafficking
   as offence, 88, 174
   organized crime, 163, 167, 175
   penalties, 172–173
   regulation of prescriptions, 170–171
training, 51–52
TUEs (therapeutic use exemptions)
   about, 56–57
   doping violations and, 77
   drugs permitted with, 44, 48–49
   issuing questionable, 207–208
   levels of substances and, 171
Turarbek, Jamilya, 83
Turin Winter Olympics (2006)
   Austrian cross-country skiing team, 72
   hematocrit levels at, 71
   media view of NHL doping, 151
20/20 television program, 88

U

UCI (Union Cycliste Internationale)
   conclusions on drug use, 202
   exposure of doping and, 92
   fight against doping, 234
   investigation of EPO allegations, 197–201
   media and, 123
   reaction to EPO allegations, 191–194
   Spanish doping investigation, 230
Ukraine, 175
UNESCO International Convention Against Doping in Sport
   creation of, 101–103
   effect on unethical professionals, 117, 208
   fight against trafficking and, 173–174
   importance of, 224
   ratification of, 227
   values of, 39
United States
   attitude towards professional sports, 122
   drug use laws, 75–77
   government response to doping, 127–128
   independent drug agency, 130
urine, manipulation of, 45, 46, 68, 85
US Congress, 124, 132–133, 148, 159–160, 226
US Constitution, 108, 111

INDEX

US Drug Enforcement Agency (DEA), 172–173
USADA (US Anti-Doping Agency)
 as agency responsible, 130
 Gatlin case, 235–236
 Lund case, 82
 Montgomery case, 86–87
USATF (USA Track & Field), 96, 235–236
USOC (United States Olympic Committee), 123, 136, 235

V

values
 society influence on, 32–33
 in sports, 10–11
 support of, 16
Vandenbroucke, Frank, 83
Verbruggen, Hein, 123, 198, 199, 202
veterinary medicine, 172
violations, 50, 77
 See also specific individuals
violence, 210–211
Voynov, Sergei, 83
Vrijman, Emile, 197, 199–201

W

WADA (World Anti-Doping Agency). *See* World Anti-Doping Agency
Warne, Shane, 80–81
White, Kelli, 56–61, 65, 87, 205
whizzinators, 68
WHO (World Health Organization), 165, 173
Williams, Ricky, 68
winning, 19–20, 27
Women's Tennis Association (WTA), 158
World Anti-Doping Agency (WADA)
 baseball and, 131
 blood doping investigation, 72–73, 77
 blood doping meeting, 71
 collaboration with pharmaceutical companies, 167–169
 criticism of efforts, 204
 development of Banned List, 40
 development of code, 97–98
 education programs, 219–220
 EPO investigation, 190–191, 198, 199–200
 gene doping conferences, 181–183, 185–186
 mission of, 15
 NBA audit, 143–144
 need for improvement, 61
 NFL discussions with, 139–140
 objectives, 94–95
 origin of, 91, 93–94
 research funds, 216–217, 223
 role of, 16, 103, 173–174, 225, 228
 UNESCO convention and, 101–103
World Anti-Doping Code
 adoption of, 99–101
 development of, 97–98, 112
 evidence for, 88
 FIFA and, 153–155
 importance of, 224
 NFL and, 140
 professional sports and, 160
 UNESCO convention and, 101–103
 values of, 39
World Baseball Classic, 131
World Championships Paris (2003), 56–57
World Conference on Doping in Sport, 98
World Cup (soccer), 152–153, 155, 156
World Health Organization (WHO), 165, 173
WTA (Women's Tennis Association), 158

Z

Zanette, Denis, 4
Zanoli, Michel, 4
ZDF television network, 234

362.29
POU

Pound, Richard W

Inside dope : how drugs are
the biggest threat to sports,
CYPRESS WOODS HS LIBRARY

26.95   12/06

DATE DUE			